The essays here expand the boundaries of psychoanalysis, applying its principles to social problems and intelligent activism while aptly demonstrating the profound applicability of our field to the socio-cultural milieu. A broad spectrum of mass trauma—including but not limited to the Holocaust, Hurricane Katrina, and September 11th—is attended to by courageous analysts who understand that their vocation must move them beyond the office walls. In the alternative tradition of Harry Stack Sullivan and Robert J. Lifton, this powerful and highly recommended volume importantly reminds us that psychoanalytic principles and practice can and should reach far outside the usual clinical frame.

—**Danielle Knafo**, author, *Living with Terror, Working with Trauma: A Clinician's Handbook*

Psychoanalysis, Trauma, and Community is essential reading for all citizen-psychoanalysts, as we meet a critical juncture in history. Confronting the effects of global violence, hatred, poverty, and oppression, we are being called by social justice. How do we apply analytic premises outside the office? The authors in this volume re-frame analytic theory, offering us a compelling guide and source of inspiration and hope.

—**Sue Grand**, NYU Postdoctoral Program in Psychotherapy and Psychoanalysis; faculty, National Institute for the Psychotherapies; faculty, the Mitchell Center for Relational Psychoanalysis and visiting scholar, the Psychoanalytic Institute of Northern California

Psychoanalysis, Trauma, and Community

Bringing together a group of eminent contributors, this volume considers how psychoanalysis may best be expanded to offer help in social and community settings and in response to disasters, wars, and serious social issues. It provides clear clinical guidance and clinical examples of how best to work psychoanalytically in a wide variety of non-traditional ways. The innovative work featured includes taking testimony, in-situ interviewing, documentary film-making, social activism, ethnic and political conflict mediation, on-site workshops as well as direct clinical interventions. The reader is taken from the Holocaust, Hiroshima and the Vietnam War to the Balkan Wars and Palestinian-Israeli conflict, from the political violence of the disappeared in Argentina to the devastation wrought by Hurricane Katrina, and from chronic conditions of poverty in India to racism in the post-Jim Crow South.

Judith L. Alpert, Ph.D., is Professor and Clinical Consultant at New York University's Postdoctoral Program in Psychotherapy and Psychoanalysis. She is also Professor of Applied Psychology and former Co-Director of the Trauma and Violence Transdisciplinary Studies Program at NYU. She maintains a private practice in New York City.

Elizabeth R. Goren, Ph.D., is faculty in the New York University Postdoctoral Program in Psychotherapy and Psychoanalysis. She is the author of numerous articles and of *Beyond the Reach of Ladders* (Open Gate Press, 2011). She is in private practice in New York City.

Relational Perspectives Book Series

Lewis Aron and Adrienne Harris, Series Editors

The Relational Perspectives Book Series (RPBS) publishes books that grow out of or contribute to the relational tradition in contemporary psychoanalysis. The term *relational psychoanalysis* was first used by Greenberg and Mitchell[1] to bridge the traditions of interpersonal relations, as developed within interpersonal psychoanalysis and object relations, as developed within contemporary British theory. But, under the seminal work of the late Stephen A. Mitchell, the term *relational psychoanalysis* grew and began to accrue to itself many other influences and developments. Various tributaries—interpersonal psychoanalysis, object relations theory, self psychology, empirical infancy research, and elements of contemporary Freudian and Kleinian thought—flow into this tradition, which understands relational configurations between self and others, both real and fantasied, as the primary subject of psychoanalytic investigation.

We refer to the relational tradition, rather than to a relational school, to highlight that we are identifying a trend, a tendency within contemporary psychoanalysis, not a more formally organized or coherent school or system of beliefs. Our use of the term *relational* signifies a dimension of theory and practice that has become salient across the wide spectrum of contemporary psychoanalysis. Now under the editorial supervision of Lewis Aron and Adrienne Harris, with the assistance of Associate Editors Steven Kuchuck and Eyal Rozmarin, the Relational Perspectives Book Series originated in 1990 under the editorial eye of the late Stephen A. Mitchell. Mitchell was the most prolific and influential of the originators of the relational tradition. Committed to dialogue among psychoanalysts, he abhorred the authoritarianism that dictated adherence to a rigid set of beliefs or technical restrictions. He championed open discussion, comparative and integrative approaches, and promoted new voices across the generations.

Included in the Relational Perspectives Book Series are authors and works that come from within the relational tradition, extend and develop that tradition, as well as works that critique relational approaches or compare and contrast it with alternative points of view. The series includes our most distinguished senior psychoanalysts, along with younger contributors who bring fresh vision. A full list of titles in this series is available at https://www.routledge.com/series/LEARPBS.

1 Greenberg, J. & Mitchell, S. (1983). *Object relations in psychoanalytic theory*. Cambridge, MA: Harvard University Press.

Psychoanalysis, Trauma, and Community

History and Contemporary Reappraisals

Edited by Judith L. Alpert and Elizabeth R. Goren

Routledge
Taylor & Francis Group
LONDON AND NEW YORK

First published 2017
by Routledge
2 Park Square, Milton Park, Abingdon, Oxon OX14 4RN

and by Routledge
711 Third Avenue, New York, NY 10017

Routledge is an imprint of the Taylor & Francis Group, an informa business

British Library Cataloguing-in-Publication Data
A catalogue record for this book is available from the British Library

Library of Congress Cataloging-in-Publication Data
Names: Alpert, Judith L., editor. | Goren, Elizabeth, 1949– editor.
Title: Psychoanalysis, trauma, and community: history and contemporary reappraisals / edited by Judith L. Alpert and Elizabeth R. Goren.
Description: Abingdon, Oxon; New York, NY: Routledge, 2017. | Includes bibliographical references and index.
Identifiers: LCCN 2016022884 | ISBN 9781138928220 (hardback: alk. paper) | ISBN 9781138928237 (pbk.: alk. paper) | ISBN 9781315681948 (e-book: alk. paper)
Subjects: LCSH: Community psychology. | Psychic trauma—Treatment. | Disasters—Psychological aspects. | Psychotherapy. | Community mental health services.
Classification: LCC RA790.55 .P79 2017 | DDC 616.89/14—dc23
LC record available at https://lccn.loc.gov/2016022884

ISBN: 978-1-138-92822-0 (hbk)
ISBN: 978-1-138-92823-7 (pbk)
ISBN: 978-1-315-68194-8 (ebk)

Typeset in Times New Roman
by codeMantra

All the contributors to this book are working to make the world a better place.

The Editors dedicate this book to our grandchildren:
Owen Max Genauer
Sia Alpert Laddis
Ben Alpert Laddis
Jake Alpert Laddis

Contents

Foreword

Nina K. Thomas

A survivor of the Holocaust, testifying at the trial of a former Nazi official said: "We have been survivors. We hope to become living people" (Dembour and Haslam, 1994). The process of becoming a living person, someone who inhabits a living present, occurs within the context of being able to have the resonating presence of another actively engage with the narrative as it unfolds. It involves acknowledgement and recognition as can only occur when we as psychoanalysts bring our close attunement to those with whom we work, mindful of our bodies as well as our minds. The dangers inherent in doing so for both participants have been detailed by a number of writers in our field including those whose work appears here. Like them, for the past thirty years I have worked in firehouses, refugee camps in post-war countries, social service agencies in the United States and abroad, talked to asylum seekers, exiles, and survivors of natural disasters. These are some of the kinds of work many of my colleagues regularly do in the course of addressing mind-numbing horrors of traumatic events that distort the worlds of those who survive. It is far from the scheduled consultation hour of private practice with its clear boundaries of space and time that provide comfort and safety. In working in such settings we are forced to adapt to the atmosphere in which we are embedded but not to alter the quality of listening we bring.

It is uncommon for psychoanalysts to enter into the aftermath of severe traumas, be those natural disasters, ethnic conflict, or the aftermath of war or racial violence. Yet it is precisely those experiences and the lessons learned from them that form the fabric of this book. Having worked in most of these settings I do not call what I did "psychoanalysis." Rather, I, like those of my colleagues whose work follows in this volume, have brought my psychoanalytic way of relating and thinking to what I term these "extra-analytic" settings. Laub and also Lifton are rightly considered the contemporary progenitors of the social activist psychoanalytic turn. Their work presented here provides robust example of the importance of the analyst in non-traditional settings who serves as "witness" to history.

In a place filled with trauma all of us are affected, sometimes together, sometimes separately. Working with trauma has the power to precipitate traumatic reactions in us all, not only those who are direct survivors of the many circumstances that may produce traumatic results. The chapters in this volume provide instances of exactly that effect. Our exposure to the trauma narratives of those to whom we consult destabilizes the denial we unconsciously maintain and that is necessary for living. We can hardly hold onto an ongoing awareness of danger lurking around every corner, of the threat of violence coming at us unexpectedly and yet for which we need to be prepared. At the same time, those with whom our authors have worked—veterans (Bassin), survivors of disaster (Wagner; Boulanger), survivors of political violence and repression (Laub; Hollander), victims of social and racial injustice (Ainslie; Roth) endure just such ongoing mindfulness of danger, threat, or renewed traumatic potential. To work with such realities as the authors in this volume have and continue to do, changes us. We continually risk being traumatized ourselves by the empathic attunement we must maintain if we are truly to listen in such settings as are described in this volume. And, as Boulanger points out (this volume), when we share the trauma survived with those with whom we work, it is no longer vicarious traumatization we endure. Rather we are "thrown into the looking glass world of shared trauma, where [our] own experiences ... reactions to them, ... self-doubts, fears and terrors mirror [our] patients' own and are reflected back in ways that are deeply disturbing" (p. 85).

What constitutes the "psychoanalytic" in the work the contributors to this volume describe is the self-reflectiveness, the processing of multiple threads, as well as the careful attention to our own and others' reactions, thoughts to the extent that we can have them, feelings; all part of our presence in such non-traditional contexts. In their introduction Alpert, Goren, and Rihm offer a moving example of applying their psychoanalytic sensibility in an educational setting. They invite two students who view one another as "enemies" to work together to fulfill a class assignment. Their creative approach to bridging difference and hostility is an example of the kind of dialogic problem solving that others have applied in order to restore an awareness of the humanity and suffering of the "other," one that emerges out of their understanding of psychoanalytic processes at play in situations of conflict.

Survivors, whether rescue worker, victim, survivor, or community, invite us to co-create their narrative of survival. In so doing we are engaged in what is essentially psychoanalytic. As we would in private practice, we must be alert to the affective changes within the narrator whether verbally or physically manifest. And we must also attend to how the telling may cause reliving the experiences not as something from the past but as something occurring in the very moment of speech; neither distant in time nor place. We need to be alert to our own lapses of attunement when the narrative becomes beyond the reach of our willingness to know. Allowing ourselves to deeply know, not merely "understand," changes us.

What I mean by knowing is a body-based attentiveness as well as reflectiveness to how my mind attends or distances from the moments of being with the people with whom I work. When do the red flags, the hair on the back of my neck, the shiver down my spine occur? How does my interviewee, group, relief worker, colleague respond to the sights, sounds, smells that surround us? The core of psychoanalysis lies in such attention to both the other and ourselves.

The events of our current times make stunningly clear how much psychological interventions are invaluable in the face of socio-psychological horrors occurring throughout our world. One glance at a newspaper or Internet news makes this abundantly obvious to those of us who would attend to the blistering, soul-destroying events wrought by natural or human-made occurrences. We who are psychoanalysts are called upon to provide our expertise in sensitively attuned moments to those whose lives have been so fundamentally altered by war, racial and social injustice, or structurally created economic disparities in housing, health care, or mental health services.

It is commonplace for the general public to think of psychoanalysis, if they wonder about it at all, as aptly characterized in the staple of *The New Yorker* cartoons. Someone is lying on a couch behind which is seated a bearded man, the stereotypical Freud. While often witty, more often such cartoons trivialize what occurs between patient and analyst. If popular notions of psychoanalysis are that it is "stale, pale, and male," that characterization is roundly challenged by the courageous and groundbreaking work of the authors in this book whose dedication to addressing the needs of the underserved, the marginalized, and those threatened regularly by the circumstances of their lives.

The psychoanalyst creates a "holding environment," a place in which safety is created by the quality of engagement between the analyst and the participant or participants. That engagement involves a resonating presence which itself acknowledges the other's experience. Speaking to a skilled and attuned listener, the patient has the opportunity to hear herself recount whatever experiences, feelings, and thoughts occupy or more often preoccupy her.

The chapters in this volume detail the application of psychoanalytic approaches by experienced and dedicated clinicians in an array of "extra-analytic" settings. They serve as models for those who share the commitment to the value and efficacy of that which is psychoanalytic and empower them to take it to the streets.

Reference

Dembour, M.B. and Haslam, E. Victim witnesses at war crimes tribunals. *European Journal of International Law*, 2004. 15 (1) pp. 155–177, n. 11, p. 154.

Notes on contributors

Ricardo C. Ainslie, Ph.D., is a psychologist–psychoanalyst who teaches at the University of Texas at Austin. His research involves using books, documentary films, and photographic exhibits to describe and reflect upon social and cultural issues in communities, especially those involving racial/ethnic conflict and violence. He also has a private practice where he sees adult patients in psychotherapy and psychoanalysis.

Judith L. Alpert, Ph.D., is Professor and Clinical Consultant at New York University's Postdoctoral Program in Psychotherapy and Psychoanalysis. She is also Professor of Applied Psychology and former Co-Director of the Trauma and Violence Transdisciplinary Studies Program at NYU. She maintains a private practice in New York City.

Neil Altman, Ph.D., is faculty at the William Alanson White Institute and an Honorary Member of the William Alanson White Society. He is also Visiting Professor at the Ambedkar University of Delhi, India, and Editor Emeritus at *Psychoanalytic Dialogues: The International Journal of Relational Perspectives*.

Lewis Aron, Ph.D., is the Director of the NYU Postdoctoral Program in Psychotherapy and Psychoanalysis. He has served as President of the Division of Psychoanalysis (39) of the American Psychological Association (APA) and was founding President of the International Association for Relational Psychoanalysis and Psychotherapy (IARPP). He is the author of *A Meeting of Minds*, and most recently with Karen Starr of *A Psychotherapy for the People: Toward a Progressive Psychoanalysis*.

Donna Bassin, Ph.D., is an author, artist, filmmaker, psychoanalyst, and veterans' advocate. She is an Adjunct Clinical Assistant Professor at the NYU Postdoctoral Program in Psychotherapy and Psychoanalysis. She has published books, articles, and reviews. She maintains a private practice in New York City.

Ghislaine Boulanger, Ph.D., is a member of the Relational faculty at NYU Postdoctoral Program in Psychotherapy and Psychoanalysis, the President of the Section for Applied Clinical Psychoanalysis of the Division of Psychoanalysis of the APA, and a member of the editorial boards of *The International Journal of Applied Psychoanalytic Studies* and *Division/Review*. Since the publication of her book, *Wounded by Reality: Understanding and Treating Adult Onset Trauma*, she has taught and published extensively on the psychodynamic dilemmas facing adults who have survived violent and life-threatening events and the clinicians who work with them. In 2008, at the invitation of the New Orleans Birmingham Psychoanalytic Center, she began visiting New Orleans regularly to speak with local clinicians about the impact of Hurricane Katrina on their lives and their practices.

Mary-Joan Gerson, Ph.D., ABPP, is an Adjunct Clinical Professor, Consultant, and was the Director of the Advanced Specialization in Couple and Family Therapy at the NYU Postdoctoral Program in Psychotherapy and Psychoanalysis. She is a Supervisor at the National Institute for the Psychotherapies and is the Founding President of Section VIII, Couples and Family Therapy, of Division 39. She is the author of numerous journal articles and book chapters focused on the integration of psychoanalytic, family systemic and attachment theory, including a full length book, *The Embedded Self: An Integrative Psychodynamic and Systemic Perspective on Couple and Family Therapy* (Routledge Press, 2009, 2nd edition), as well as many publications about chronic illness, adult development, and psychoanalytic activism.

Elizabeth R. Goren, Ph.D., is faculty in the New York University Postdoctoral Program in Psychotherapy and Psychoanalysis. She is the author of numerous articles and of *Beyond the Reach of Ladders* (Open Gate Press, 2011). She is in private practice in New York City.

Elizabeth Hegeman, Ph.D., has been Professor at John Jay College of Criminal Justice–City University New York (CUNY) for forty-nine years; she is on the faculty, training analyst and supervising analyst at W.A. White Institute, and faculty at NYU Postdoctoral Program in

Psychoanalysis and Manhattan Institute for Psychoanalysis. She is a member of the Editorial Board of *Contemporary Psychoanalysis* and has written about trauma, dissociation, and multiple self-states. With Michael Stocker she co-authored *Valuing Emotions*. Her most recent research and publication is on ethnic syndromes which involve primitive self-states and dissociative defenses. She has been in private practice for forty-two years.

Nancy Caro Hollander, Ph.D., is a research psychoanalyst in private practice in Oakland, California, and a faculty member of the Psychoanalytic Institute of Northern California. She is President of Psychoanalysis for Social Responsibility, Section 9 of Division 39, APA, and Professor Emerita of Latin American history, California State University. Over the past three decades, she has published her work on social psychoanalysis in national and international journals and is co-editor and contributor (with Lynne Layton and Susan Gutwill) of *Psychoanalysis, Class and Politics: Encounters in the Clinical Setting* (Routledge, 2007) and author of *Uprooted Minds: Surviving the Politics of Terror in the Americas* (Routledge, 2010).

Alison Lake, M.A., L.P., holds a Masters in Anthropology from Princeton University and is a licensed psychoanalyst. She works as a consulting project director in suicide prevention research, and as a psychoanalytic psychotherapist in private practice.

Dori Laub, M.D., was born in Cernauti, Romania, on June 8, 1937. He is currently a practicing psychoanalyst in New Haven, Connecticut, who works primarily with victims of massive psychic trauma and with their children. He is Clinical Professor of Psychiatry at the Yale University School of Medicine and co-founder of the Fortunoff Video Archive for Holocaust Testimonies.

Andrea Rihm, M.A., Ph.D., is an art therapist and clinical psychologist. She works in private practice and is part of the Interdisciplinary Laboratory of Studies on Subjectivity and Social Change in Santiago, Chile. Her interests revolve around art therapy and psychoanalysis, trauma, and immigration.

Judy Roth, Ph.D., is a clinical psychologist/psychoanalyst and Associate Medical Professor and Supervisor at CUNY. She is co-founder of

Born Equal, a taskforce of scholar–practitioners working to understand the psychological realities for families living with political violence in Israel and Palestine (http://bornequal.net). She is co-chair of the Global Psychosocial Network, a project of Psychologists for Social Responsibility, providing psychosocial support for those engaged in humanitarian work in conflict zones (http://www.globalpsychosocialnetwork.org). Relevant writing includes: "Crows on the cradles: Palestinian mothers at a frontline vortex." Her clinical interests involve the existential junctures of adult development; mothering across the lifespan; and the transmission of social trauma and resilience. She maintains a diverse private practice.

Vamik D. Volkan, M.D., DLFAPA, FACPsa, is Emeritus Professor of Psychiatry at the University of Virginia, Charlottesville, Virginia, and Emeritus Training and Supervising Analyst at the Washington Psychoanalytic Institute, Washington, D.C. He holds Honorary Doctorate degrees from the University of Eastern Finland, Finland, from Ankara University, Turkey, and Eastern European Psychoanalytic Institute, Russia. He is the President of the International Dialogue Initiative and a former President of the Turkish–American Neuropsychiatric Society, the International Society of Political Psychology, the Virginia Psychoanalytic Society, and the American College of Psychoanalysts.

Laurel Bass Wagner, Ph.D., is a Clinical Professor of Psychology at the University of Texas Southwestern Medical Center at Dallas and a past-President of the Division of Psychoanalysis (Division 39) of the American Psychological Association. She was the founding chairperson of the Disaster Response Team for the Dallas Psychological Association in the late 1980s. Since then she has responded to numerous disasters, including mass shootings, airplane crashes, and natural disasters.

Introduction: Expanding our analytic identity

The inclusion of a larger social perspective

Judith L. Alpert, Elizabeth R. Goren, and Andrea Rihm

It was early in the fall semester, around September 11, 2002. The event took place in a graduate-level trauma course. The professor, a psychoanalyst, referred to the *terrorists* who flew their planes into the Twin Towers. An Arab student raised her hand and corrected the professor, informing her that the pilots were not terrorists. When the professor asked what they were, Abia, the student, responded: "freedom fighters." A painful noise in response to this statement came from an Israeli student seated behind the Arab student. This is how the semester began.

While there are many ways the professor could have responded to the situation, this is what the professor did. She indicated that the course did not focus on politics and that she was not interested in passing the hot potato of blame. Rather, she indicated that the course focus was on trauma and the horrific impact of war and other human-made events.

Seismic upheavals clearly lay ahead. Several weeks later Abia approached the professor and asked for an appointment. When the instructor asked what she wanted to talk about, the response was piercing and powerful: "I want to talk about my hatred of you."

Professor and student met. In fact, they met many times over the course of the semester. Abia indicated that she hated the professor because she was a Jewess who supported Israelis and, therefore, was anti-Palestinian. Over time, it became clear that Abia had no basis for saying this. It was just her supposition. As they continued to talk, Abia revealed that she hated all Jewish people as well as all Israelis and was sure that "Jewish" was the primary focus and identity of all Jews. The professor pointed out that gender rather than religion comprised her primary identity. Abia was shocked.

Things shifted after this. Abia was encouraged to answer questions and think about issues from two self-states: (1) the self-state of a Palestinian and (2) the self-state of a female. Abia's Palestinian voice spoke of hate, retaliation, Hamas, Fatach, Intifada, violent conflict, and destruction. Abia's female voice spoke of traditional distribution of power, closed doors, iron gates, confinement, invisibility, relinquishing rights, subservience, servitude, and of a desire for modernization as an antidote to extremism.

Over time Abia was encouraged to consider reaching out and, possibly, writing a course paper with Golda, the Israeli student. With the professor present, Abia and Golda discussed the possibility of co-writing a paper on their experience of war in their country. They met over several weeks. Finally both students agreed to write a paper together: Each would pose questions that the other would answer. These answers, once compiled into one paper, would satisfy the course assignment. The professor would be on call as needed to help them to complete this project and to deal with the difficulties and tensions encountered between and within them.

The two students, one with a family living in Gaza among the airstrikes and relentless sounds of earthquake-like explosions, Israeli Apache helicopters, and F-16s flying overhead, and the other, with an Israeli family living among Hezbollah missiles, hopes of ceasefires, and belief in right to defend, wrote an honest, heart-wrenching paper which they read to the class. Nothing would ever be the same for all those present.

You may wonder why we are including this example in a chapter on psychoanalysis outside the office? While this is a confabulated story drawn from several similar events that occurred while teaching, the alterations do not diminish understanding about psychoanalysts providing psychoanalytically informed interventions outside the office. The case illustrates one uncharacteristic way in which a psychoanalyst applied psychoanalytically oriented thinking and therapeutic practices to a social issue outside the consulting room.

We know that many psychoanalysts today are busy bringing the analytic perspective and clinical skills into many contexts far beyond the traditional office setting so embedded in the analytic identity, and some even taking psychoanalysis even beyond strictly defined therapeutic settings. Further, we propose that the field, with our understanding of the human psyche, interpersonal relationships, and group dynamics, can make an important contribution to pressing social and world problems and to the welfare and healing of communities. Variously referred to as "applied psychoanalysis" or "psychoanalysis in community" or "taking psychoanalysis out of the office," the chapters in this book illustrate the range of issues and types of interventions that this kind of work can entail. Our interest here is in looking at psychoanalytic applications beyond conventional clinical settings.

Not surprisingly, analytic interventions in the community typically involve working with trauma at the individual, group, and collective level, and run the gamut from acute and massive social trauma like disasters, ongoing states of terrorism and war to chronic conditions of poverty, illness, and immigration. Psychoanalytically informed interventions also take place as a ripple effect of these issues such as in the classroom situation just described. As the articles in this book demonstrate, these interventions address prejudice, interpersonal and group tensions, conflict and social distress related to racial, class, ethnic, and nationalistic issues.

Rationale for expanding analytic identity and mission

Two fundamental questions lie behind the idea of expanding the reach of psychoanalysis beyond the individual and the office. Is it appropriate or necessary for us to move beyond a mission of individual change through the practice of therapy? A related question is whether we have the knowledge and skills to take on this challenge. To both of these questions we say: yes, and we hope that the chapters in this book will inspire you to join us in this effort.

A number of factors have combined to make consideration of expanding psychoanalytic interventions and the role of analysts a timely matter. A few of the most salient issues include changes in broader culture, such as conceptions and modes of delivery of mental health services, the marginalization of psychoanalysis within psychology and in the public eye, and the liberalization of theory and practice within the discipline of psychoanalysis itself. From our recent past, we mark 9/11 as a major turning point for psychoanalysts, as for Americans in general. The more recent work featured in this volume by Neil Altman, Ricardo Ainslie, Laurie Wagner, Nancy Hollander, Judy Roth, Lew Aron, Donna Bassin, Vamik Volkan, Mary-Joan Gerson, Elizabeth Hegeman, and Ghislaine Boulanger reflect these cultural changes in the field and in society. The work of early leaders like Robert Jay Lifton, whose interview appears in this volume, and Dori Laub and the chapter by Lewis Aron show how social activism and non-traditional applications of psychoanalysis were being made before this historic moment. The fifteen years since 9/11 have been characterized by a state of terrorism, wars, and economic depression, giving rise to increased value on volunteerism and a renewed commitment to public service.

Social advocacy and justice, though a longstanding mission for mental health organizations, appears to have become the issue of the day. Both the American Psychoanalytic Association and the American Psychological Association have undertaken initiatives on a range of social issues like immigration, multicultural diversity, and sexuality. Within the American Psychoanalytic Association, for example, there is a Community and Society Committee whose mission statement emphasizes the role and responsibility that psychoanalysts have in addressing the complex issues and problems created by external reality. Similarly one section within the American Psychological Association's Division of Psychoanalysis (Section IX Division 39), Psychoanalysis for Social Responsibility, is specifically dedicated to bringing a psychoanalytic perspective to contemporary social issues such as human rights, race relations, education, poverty, and violence. Its mission is to promote the accessibility of psychoanalytically oriented clinical service to underserved groups of people, and to the development of theory and technique geared to the goal of expanding the cultural and socio-economic usefulness of psychoanalytic treatment. Additionally, until recently there was a committee in the Division of Psychoanalysis, American Psychological Association titled "Psychoanalysis and Community Committee," which was chaired by Judie Alpert and Mary-Joan Gerson. It had the mandate of expanding the reach of psychoanalysis into the community. While this committee no longer exists, other sections of the association have taken up the focus.

Yet another example: both the American Psychoanalytic Association and the American Psychological Association have taken and continue to take a definitive stand against any of its members participating in torture. Finally, in her presidential address to the American Psychoanalytic Association, Gourguechon (2011) declared a public health crisis in the culture, which she describes as being a "national emergency of superficiality."

It is our contention that this powerful innovative form of psychoanalysis has received less attention and, as a result, less respect than it deserves. In support of Bernard and Kelly's (1998) claim that social problems such as racism, poverty, or war have a bearing on mental health and illness, we believe that we have a responsibility as analysts to reflect on these issues and consider expanding our analytic identity and important function in contributing to improving the welfare of the world and its inhabitants.

History

If applied psychoanalysis is so crucial, why has it not received more attention? We think that the oft-cited expression "psychoanalysis and the couch" captures the deeply entrenched image of psychoanalysis and resistance to change. Our patients, the public, even psychoanalysts, tend to think of our work as a form of psychotherapy in the private setting of the office. As a result, the vast majority of psychoanalytic literature and training, reflective of our very psychoanalytic identity, has typically focused on conventional one-on-one treatment, or at most, group therapy. While we tend to think of the kind of work highlighted in this volume as untraditional or unconventional, there have always been analysts who have innovatively taken psychoanalytic principles and therapeutic practices outside the office setting. Moreover, throughout the past 120 years, the need to reconceptualize, redefine, and broaden professional roles and practices has been a recursive one, not only for psychoanalysts, but for psychiatrists and psychologists as well. Nonetheless, somehow, these efforts have not made it sufficiently to psychoanalysis's mainstream.

Indeed, our present analytic identity is much narrower than some of our founding fathers and mothers envisioned it to be. Many of our psychoanalytic forerunners yearned to make psychoanalysis available outside the consulting room and to the general public, starting with Freud himself. As Elizabeth Danto (2005) has stressed, even if Freud's theory might have aimed to be scientific and ahistorical, his clinical practice certainly was not. He would regularly see patients at the Vienna free clinic and, in 1918, at the Fifth International Congress in Budapest, he summoned psychoanalysts to develop free out-patient clinics, stating that "the poor man should have just as much right to assistance for his mind as he now has to the life-saving help offered by surgery" (cited in Danto, 2005, p. 1). Freud also wanted to see psychoanalysis applied to education and the rearing of the next generation, as he mentioned in *Explanations, Applications and Orientations* (Freud, 1933). As indicated by Aron and Starr (2013), psychoanalytic identity—as a "soft assembly" (Harris, 2005)—is contingent and could have followed a number of different trajectories. In fact, Twemlow and Parens (2006) have advanced the view that Freud's main legacy might lie beyond the couch and actually involve the role of psychoanalysis in community and social problems.

Thus, social activism, intimately involved with the dedicated extension of psychoanalysis beyond the consulting room, has its roots in the earliest days of psychoanalysis, with the free clinics established throughout Europe in the 1920s and 1930s. Altman (1995), Sklarew, Twemlow, and Wilkinson (2004), Twemlow (2004), and Danto (2005) provide reviews of this history.

The Second World War changed history and, with it, the course and development of psychoanalysis and all mental health professions too. The reality of war, death, and their ensuing social problems became unavoidable protagonists of culture (Sarason et al., 1966). As Phillips (1988) noted, Winnicott was known for highlighting the importance of external reality in the psychoanalytic situation. At the British Psychoanalytic Society meeting that took place during the Second World War, Winnicott pointed out to the group that it was ignoring the reality that bombs were dropping. The acknowledgment of both external reality and consulting room reality was also key for Melitta Schmideberg (1942), Melanie Klein's daughter. She recognized the traumatic external wartime truth as well as the common fears of patient and analyst sharing a life-threatening situation.

With them, a number of analysts, in Europe, continued their commitment to take psychoanalysis outside the consulting room and into institutions that played a major role in social life. Take Anna Freud for example. She consulted and collaborated with non-analytic professionals about child development, laid down a model for child analysts, and supported the training of candidates in applied psychoanalysis (A. Freud, 1971). She was not alone.

The Tavistock Institute of Human Relations, founded in the 1940s, had a socio-psychological approach, and sought ways to apply psychoanalytic concepts to settings different than individual psychotherapy, particularly to group and organizational life. They focused on how unconscious processes were enacted in these contexts. An example is the work of Isabel Menzies (1960) who considered social defenses against anxiety. Her approach continues to be utilized today (e.g., Canham, 2001; Stein, 2004), and has expanded to the application of analytic concepts to organizational contexts, by consultants and coaches in the workplace. Its popularity is evidenced by the fact that a recent issue of *Psychoanalytic Dialogues*

(Vol. 22, 2012) was devoted to psychoanalysis and organizations. In that issue, Aron (2012) acknowledged the influence of Wilfred Bion (1961, 1967) to this area of the field's development.

In the United States, and particularly in the field of mental health, the impact of the Second World War materialized through several confluent paths. On one hand, it meant the arrival of a significant number of European analyst émigrés who reshaped the development and teaching of psychoanalysis. On the other, it boosted the development of clinical psychology as a distinct field as well as the reconceptualization of mental health.

According to Sarason et al. (1966), before the Second World War there were no professional training programs for clinical psychology in the United States. American psychology was "academic" in its orientation and anti-clinical. Thus, in order to train new professionals who could respond to the aftermath of the Second World War, clinical psychology had to depend on other mental health disciplines, especially psychiatry. But, as Sarason (1995) recapitulates, psychiatry was not fully prepared to deal with the clinical aspects of psychiatric issues related directly or indirectly to war experiences. In this context, psychoanalysis stood out as a model and became mainstream within psychiatry departments for the first time. Thus, psychoanalysis experienced a number of years of unusual calm, as noted by Aron and Starr (2013). Nonetheless, being part of the mainstream also exposed psychoanalysis to greater criticism. Beginning in the 1960s, psychoanalysis as a theory and a practice came to be critically scrutinized (Sarason, 1995).

Psychoanalysis was not the only field under examination. Psychiatry was also under scrutiny as many clinical psychologists were realizing the constraints entailed by a medical model of intervention. Within the medical model, patients were seen in doctor's offices. Thus, the medical model limited the range of human problems dealt with and narrowed the potential for intervention around social problems. Also, Albee (1970) posited that by adopting psychiatric explanations of sickness, clinical psychology might have been sustaining rather than challenging cultural forces that delayed the needed social changes necessary to prevent emotional problems. Thus, there was a growing a sense of dissatisfaction with the professional identity among some clinicians. This dissatisfaction led some professionals to a shift in focus from the individual to the community (Albee, 1970; Sarason et al., 1966).

Clinical psychologists were not alone in this effort. On the contrary, in the second half of the twentieth century, with its upheavals and transformations, it became increasingly difficult for psychoanalysts, psychiatrists, and social workers to ignore a consideration of the impact of social issues on subjectivity, psychic life and, therefore, on clinical practice.

Meanwhile, within the American psychoanalytic movement the ideals of social change and professional activism became a defining focus and mission of the emerging Cultural and Interpersonal Schools. There were influential contributions from such analysts as Horney, Sullivan, and Fromm. They contributed to psychoanalytic theory and technique as well as to our understanding of cultural forces, human nature, and individual development.

Harry Stack Sullivan conceptualized psychiatry as a field concerned with human living in its entirety, comprehending the individual, sociocultural and communal aspects of it. As he stressed:

> ...psychiatry is neither the mentally sick individual, nor the successful and unsuccessful processes that may be observed in groups and that can be studied in detached objectivity. Psychiatry, instead, is the study of processes that involve or go on between people. The field of psychiatry is the field of interpersonal relations, under any and all circumstances in which these relations exist (2012, p. 8).

Thus, from his perspective, psychiatry should engage in dialogue with psychobiology, cultural anthropology, and—especially—social psychology, to enrich its understandings (Sullivan, 1955/2001). Even more so, for psychiatry to become a *psychiatry of peoples*, he believed it should develop a better grasp of the different cultural patterns of living around the world (Sullivan, 1948/2011).

Karen Horney (1937/1999) also stressed the importance of the relation between cultural conditions and mental health. In the first pages of *The Neurotic Personality of Our Time* she clearly stated her position:

> When we focus our attention on the actual neurotic difficulties, we recognize that neuroses are generated not only by incidental individual experiences, but also by the specific cultural conditions under which we live. In fact, the cultural conditions not only lend weight and

> color to the individual experiences but in the last analysis determine their particular form (p. viii).

Thus, for Horney (1937/1999), acknowledging the importance of cultural conditions involved challenging conceptions of normality and departing from more traditional psychoanalytic interpretations of neuroses.

Erich Fromm (1955/1970) also considered normalcy and mental health as an individual problem of adjustment to a certain social order. He critically analyzed the pathology of normalcy within contemporary societies and associated it to a lifestyle that did not satisfy the profound needs of the human condition. Moreover, he argued that the crisis he perceived in psychoanalysis was related to this issue, positing that while initially psychoanalysis had offered many a space to be listened to, along its development it had failed to sufficiently transform in response to the changed human situation after the First World War. His observation was that psychoanalysis had retreated into conformism and the search for respectability, losing its most radical character. From Fromm's perspective, this transformation of theory from radical to conformist could be explained by the choice made by Freud's disciples to discontinue the more radical paths Freud had opened and, in the end, emphasize those theoretical aspects that would be deemed more acceptable. Stated differently: Fromm believed that psychoanalytic theory did not go beyond cultural restrictions because there was a conscious effort, on behalf of Freud's disciples, to present a theory which would be deemed more acceptable by the society of the time.

Departing from traditional views and despite their differences in emphasis, Sullivan, Horney, and Fromm simultaneously focused on theorizing about the societal forces that created the individual's problems, providing clinical service, consulting with public health related organizations, and through their writing and public voice, bringing their psychoanalytic perspective to the community at large.

The acknowledgment of the role of cultural conditions and forces in determining mental health was shared by a number of professionals from outside the field of psychoanalysis. The advent of effective psychopharmacology and the ensuing de-institutionalization movement marked the need to work differently with a broader group of patients, particularly those who had historically been institutionalized (Drake et al., 2003). Attuned with these new circumstances, Viola Bernard and Karl Menninger founded the field of community psychiatry. They considered social problems in the early days of de-institutionalization. At this time, Gerald Caplan (1961) delineated a proposal for preventive psychiatry and for community mental health. He understood that effective treatments should encompass clinical and administrative interventions, all with the aim of helping patients to return to their communities. Thus, Caplan envisioned an intervention model that included the reduction of potentially stressful living conditions as well as a multitude of interventions from different fields and from such domains as psychiatry, rehabilitation, and employment.

In the midst of these developments, the *Community Mental Health Act* was signed in 1963, ushering in a new stage. Beginning in 1965, numerous community mental health centers were created and funded throughout the country (Cutler, Bevilacqua & McFarland, 2003). The opening of these new spaces allowed psychoanalytically oriented professionals to work with the community and with people from the inner city (Altman, 1995).

This encounter, however, was not devoid of criticism. Analysts and other professionals raised questions regarding the training and competence of psychoanalysts to work with chronically ill patients who were in need of various services (Cutler et al., 2003). Yet, as noted by Altman (2010), it also stimulated questioning and renewal of psychoanalytic thinking regarding its application to broader social groups. At around the same time, the Conference on the Professional Preparation of Clinical Psychologists took place. According to Sarason and collaborators (1966), the conference channeled some of the controversies in the field and marked the beginning of a new professional era, one in which community mental health played a greater role.

In this regard, it is important to stress that, while there was a history of social activism within psychoanalysis, the historical record reveals that not all were in agreement that psychoanalysts should engage in psychoanalytic advocacy (Gourguechon, 2011). In fact, there was notable dissension from the American Psychoanalytic Association's Committee for the Study of Social Issues (1951).

While Sullivan, Horney, and Fromm were calling on analysts to engage in reflections on social conditions, Lawrence Kubie (1950) voiced his opposition to analysts engaging in the public arena. He noted the need for analysts to maintain anonymity and his concern that extra-analytic preoccupations would negatively impact the analyst's focus on the inner world of patients.

Thus, the appropriateness of social advocacy and community intervention has been a longstanding controversy in the field and continues to this day (see Oliner, 1996 and Twemlow, 2004 for reviews). Nevertheless, despite the folklore of psychoanalysis as a one-on-one therapeutic practice for the elite of society, and in the face of opposition within the field, many psychoanalysts engaged in work with communities in the past and they continue to do so today as the chapters in this book illustrate.

The contemporary story

The number of contemporary psychoanalysts involved in the broader mission has steadily increased over time. For some, involvement was taken on in response to recent acute traumatic situations like social and natural disasters, terrorism, and war. A growing number of analysts today devote themselves to working both in and beyond the office with populations impacted by chronic traumatic conditions of life such as poverty, illness, and immigration.

In her call for action, Gourguechon (2011) identified seven ways the "citizen" analyst can contribute to the public good: (1) psychoanalytic social commentary; (2) psychoanalytic social advocacy; (3) psychoanalysis in the community; (4) psychoanalysis of the community; (5) psychoanalytic interpretation in the academy; (6) using data to promote social change; and (7) developing theory of applying psychoanalytic thought to culture.

As the chapters in this book demonstrate, much of the work of analysts in this area crosses these distinct categories, often simultaneously including clinical interventions, conceptual elements, and social activist intent. Nonetheless the classification system is a useful framework for the work encompassed in the expanding psychoanalytic project, as you will see in our highlighting of some of the contemporary work in this area.

Psychoanalytic social commentary involves explanatory and interpretive commentary and focuses on motivation, including whenever possible, explanations of phenomena such as transference and countertransference, the unconscious, and other basic psychoanalytic concepts. One example is provided by Sandler and Alpert's (2000) consideration of a school shooting in suburban America, in which Eric Harris and Dylan Klebold raged into their Columbine, Colorado, high school and killed thirteen classmates in addition to themselves. Applying key concepts from the psychoanalytic literature, Sandler and Alpert describe how the groups' unconscious processes led to the development of particular roles for Klebold and Harris and use the concepts of projective identification, splitting, basic assumption groups, and the social defense system to develop the position that these two youths were the recipients of the group's projections and, further, that the group was complicit in developing Klebold's and Harris's role as offenders. The impact of groups in the particular developmental stage of adolescence was also considered.

The Association for the Psychoanalysis of Culture & Society (APCS), an international and interdisciplinary non-profit organization, is the ideal example of social commentary. Consider its mission statement:

> ...to promote the use of psychoanalysis for the solution of social problems. The most serious of these problems, including interpersonal, international, institutional and structural violence as well as drug abuse, irresponsible sexuality, and intolerance in its various forms, will be extremely difficult if not impossible to solve unless we address the psychological roots that are the immediate causes of these destructive behaviors.

Further, it posits

> Psychoanalysis offers the best model we have for understanding how the most basic and powerful psychological forces—love, hate, knowledge belief, meaning, identity, desire, enjoyment, fantasy—function as both causes and effects of social and cultural phenomena. The psychoanalytic investigation of culture and society thus constitutes a unique and arguably indispensable means of understanding and intervening around the psychological roots of our most serious social problems as well as understanding and promoting the psychological and social benefits that various social formations and cultural phenomena offer.

Its annual conference, the projects it promotes, and its journal, *Psychoanalysis, Culture & Society*, focus on the connection between psychoanalysis and the social world, and explores the possible roles for psychoanalysts in promoting collective justice and necessary reform.

Like much of the work and literature on this subject, the chapters in this book fall under the category of psychoanalysis *in* and *of* the community.

In addition to being community interventions they involve social commentary and might be considered forms of social advocacy. For example, Wagner writes about the multiple traumas of New Orleans residents who were forced to evacuate to a shelter in Dallas after Hurricane Katrina. She worked on site at a direct clinical level with children and their families as well as at the organizational level to develop analytically informed services and programs. Ainslie explores the differences between the White and Black communities in terms of their Texas town's history segregation and designed interventions, which potentiated airing grievances and mutual healing.

A complete review of community interventions is beyond the scope of this introduction, but one example that involves intervention in and of the community as well as social commentary is Elizabeth Goren's (2011) work with the Fire Department of New York after 9/11. She details the clinical challenges of being a therapist embedded in a firehouse. Elaborating on the nature of trauma and grief in laymen's language for accessibility to the public, she describes a series of analytically informed therapeutic strategies designed to engage men who were resistant to having an outsider brought into their world. Lastly, another kind of relevant community intervention is exemplified by Felix and Wine's (2001) work with the homeless. During the stages of outreach and engagement, they point to the utility of Winnicott's (1965/1990) holding environment, Bion's (1977) concept of the container, and Erikson's (1950) description of basic trust versus mistrust. In considering the management of transference and countertransference, they point to the utility of Kohut's self-psychology, specifically his concepts of mirroring, idealized object transferences, and the primacy of empathy. They note the value of Kernberg's work on object relations (Kernberg, 1976) and, in particular the role of primitive defenses, identity diffusion, and aggression.

Psychoanalytic interpretation in the academy involves the application of psychoanalytic ideas to literature, the arts, humanities, and the social sciences. This is a contribution to the academic and psychoanalytic literature. Space limitations do not allow us to mention all the work that has been done or is presently ongoing. We identify a few. The works of Philip Cushman (1994) and Drew Westen (2007), among many others, have broadened the scope of the psychoanalytic perspective into the areas of social, cultural, and political theory and psychoanalysis. A solid body of work by Lynn Layton (2011) and Muriel Dimen (2011) exemplify the application of psychoanalytic lens to postmodern studies, gender, and multicultural studies.

A different type of academic application is the cross-disciplinary dialogue that takes place in journals such as *Psychoanalysis, Culture & Society*, and at conferences such as the annual meeting of the APCS. Another example is the Interdisciplinary Freud Research Group, which was co-organized by Lewis Aron, Director of the Postdoctoral Program in Psychotherapy and Psychoanalysis, and Shireen Patell, former Clinical Assistant Professor and Associate Director of the Trauma and Violence Transdisciplinary Studies Program, New York University. The group consists of New York University (NYU) faculty members, graduate students, and postdoctoral students from a wide variety of academic disciplines and departments including French, German, English, Cinema Studies, Performance Studies, Applied Psychology, Media, Culture, and Communication, Gender & Sexuality, Trauma Studies, The Draper Interdisciplinary Program, the Law School, and the Postdoctoral Program in Psychotherapy and Psychoanalysis.

Gourguechon (2011) identifies *developing the theory* of applying psychoanalytic thought to culture and promoting social change. This involves the theoretical exploration of the meaning and validity of applying psychoanalytic ideas to social and cultural phenomena. *Psychoanalytic social advocacy* refers to a psychoanalyst or analytic organization taking a stand on a public issue and working toward the resolution of that issue. An example: our offering public comment, interpretations, and explanations on an issue being considered by the public with the goal of advancing our psychoanalytic way of thinking about the human mind. In this way, we contribute to an understanding of human experience.

Finally, we have psychoanalysts like Volkan (1999 a, b, c,) whose work crosses several categories, encompassing therapeutic intervention, conceptual formulations on violence and massive social trauma, and a goal of social change. Writing about international conflict, inter-ethnic strife and other large-scale problems, he takes the position that unconscious processes must be dealt with by nations and communities in order to establish truly enduring resolutions to intergenerational conflicts. Using an active-interventionist/group-focused approach, Volkan instigates dialogue between community leaders, and he works to engage participants toward the reframing of issues, questions, and solutions.

Today there is a continuum. At one end is the psychoanalyst who focuses solely on psychic reality in the consulting room. At the other is the psychoanalyst who leaves his office and works to facilitate resolution of social problems while recognizing the impact of external reality on inner lives. While few do the latter full time, theoretically it could comprise one's full practice and could necessitate specialized training.

Challenges

In 2004, Kogan posed a challenge to the field:

> At a time when war and destruction are part of everyday life, and our safety is increasingly threatened, one of the questions we Israeli analysts ask ourselves is, What is the place of psychoanalysis in such a world? Can we in good faith propose to practice psychoanalysis in situations of chronic crises, and can we, in the face of the effect of terrorism, hold on to our identities as psychoanalysts? (pp. 735–736)

A decade later, Kogan's plea for us to see the urgency of the need still rings true. Applying psychoanalysis to facilitate the resolution of social problems and healing at the community level requires technical changes, as the authors in this book discuss more fully.

As Twemlow and Parens (2006) point out in their review of the relevant literature, analysts need to be flexible and humble in their engagement. They must be prepared to give up, at times, a position of neutrality and abstinence, to use transference for purposes of influence rather than interpretation, and to accept a more limited role than they are accustomed to, meaning being a team member rather than a leader. Clearly, the psychoanalyst's bearing is different depending on whether one is working in the consulting room or in the community.

There are choices to be made and psychoanalytic technique must be reconsidered as Altman (1995, 2010) and others have indicated. In recent decades, psychoanalysis has progressively moved from a one-person theory to a two-person theory. Aron (1991) conceptualizes this shift as one where the analyst's identity, his/her whole being makes a difference for the patient. How does this change impact on the psychoanalyst's stance in contexts of community psychoanalysis? Some suggest maintaining a traditional stance, where the analyst in a group assumes the role of non-participant interpreter of group functioning. Others propose a more activist group-focused stance, focusing the intervention on actively changing how the group functions rather than on simply interpreting its underlying dynamics. Regardless of the analyst's technical stance, the community analyst depends on her psychoanalytic knowledge base for action. Examples of the latter approach are provided in Mukherjee and Alpert's (2006) consideration of community-based interventions in the acute aftermath of disaster and in Sklarew et al.'s (2004) anthology.

Working in a social context creates complexity. A two-person psychoanalytic perspective views the treatment situation as involving the analyst and the patient, with the analyst understood as a full and active member in an interaction. Altman goes beyond the two-person model (1995, 2010) and terms a model that includes a larger social perspective, a "three-person model," with the third person representing the social context. Thus, the third would lead us to attend to the analytic significance of the disaster or terrorism or the traumatic and chronic conditions of poverty unemployment, illness, and immigration relevant to the context. It may be, as A. Freud (1971) and Twemlow and Parens (2006) have suggested, that training institutes should offer education specifically geared to working in the community. The range of work covered in this volume and the unique challenges each analyst faced in reaching outside the office frame are meant to contribute to building an educational base in this area.

Chapters in this book

In addition to this introduction and a conclusion, the book is made up of four parts: (1) Receiving testimony; (2) Therapeutic encounters outside the frame; (3) Facilitating collective mourning; and (4) Psychoanalytic scholarship and activism.

The first part (Receiving testimony) includes chapters by Dori Laub and Judy Roth. Laub's work has also involved interviewing, specifically toward the taking of testimony. His work is psychoanalytically informed and makes clear that testimony is a social phenomenon, a personally meaningful and therapeutic relational experience, as well as a culturally healing process. In his chapter, he explains how, before testimony, a witness does not know what she knows of her experience of extremity. The testimonial process, in the company of an intimate and psychoanalytically astute listener, can facilitate greater consciousness and potential reckoning with frozen memories. Further, he explains how a testimonial intervention has a therapeutic effect in that it both creates a remembered past and frees up the emotional space for present living.

Roth focuses on the continuous traumas of political violence in Palestine and Israel. She reflects on experiences of people who are standing at thresholds, beginning with the experience of participants in a truth commission and then moving to the experiences of Palestinian parents and children living in the more besieged neighborhood of hostility and concludes by discussing the experiences of human rights workers and professionals who work alongside those living in these beleaguered districts. She raises many questions such as: Is witnessing in a zone of ongoing conflict a good idea and, if so, to whom is it helpful? After raising many important questions, she speaks to what clinicians can offer in these situations and what may be downsides to their offerings. She concludes by noting that listening is a privilege that changes the listener.

In the second section, "Therapeutic encounters outside the frame," Laurel Bass Wagner and Ghislaine Boulanger discuss different aspects of experience related to Hurricane Katrina. Wagner describes her experience as a first responder in the Red Cross shelters in Dallas, Texas. By means of clinical vignettes, she illustrates the mental states of survivors of Hurricane Katrina, the complicated results from the poor preparation for and response to the Katrina disaster, the appalling conditions of the shelter in New Orleans, and the relocation to shelters in Dallas. She tells the story of psychological first aid and presents case illustrations of a psychoanalytic approach to first aid disaster response at both a clinical and organizational level and she places this in theoretical context. In the next chapter, Boulanger discusses the situation in which the clinician has experienced the same or similar events as those seeking her professional help. She points out that in this situation the term "vicarious trauma" does not apply. Rather, the clinician, sharing the trauma with her patient, mirrors her patients. This was the dilemma facing local clinicians in New Orleans in the wake of Hurricane Katrina, and Boulanger considers the different phases that clinicians passed through.

While Neil Altman is not writing about Hurricane Katrina, his chapter belongs in this section as he provides information about therapeutic encounters outside the frame. He provides historical information as to how psychoanalysis came to be thought of largely as an office-based practice for an affluent, culturally specific clientele. He then considers efforts to train candidates and students in India on how to deal with cross-cultural and socio-economic divides and how to use the informality of spontaneously occurring interactions in the natural environment to illuminate unconscious interpersonal and intrapsychic dynamics. He concludes by suggesting that the mentalization fostered by psychoanalytic processing of these interactions can provide a protective element against the intergenerational transmission of trauma.

The third section, "Facilitating collective mourning," includes chapters by Ricardo C. Ainslie, Donna Bassin, and Vamik D. Volkan. Ainslie presents material from a creatively inspired clinical intervention. His interests focus on the relations between trauma and memory as well as the significance of giving voice and representation as part of the healing process. In this chapter, he describes three interrelated psychoanalytically informed interventions in a Texas community where conflict-laden residues of the Jim Crow era continue to impact on race relations.

Bassin describes her work as "an attempt to work through aspects of veterans' struggles to 'come back home,' share some of their restorative efforts in this journey, and contribute to a growing practice of psychoanalytically-minded community mental health workers, while also reflecting on my own professional changes following 9/11." She draws a conclusion through a work in progress, a warehouse-sized art installation that is a collaborative mourning space. Her chapter provides a summary of the path that led to the development of such a space.

Volkan, in this section, provides a definition of large group identity that is, according to Volkan, "sufficient to explain the power it has to influence political, economic, legal, and military initiatives and to induce seemingly irrational resistances to finding peaceful solutions to large group conflicts." Also, he describes societal responses when the "other," "who possesses a different large-group identity than the victims, humiliates, and oppresses a large group and threatens its large-group's identity." He considers the psychological effects of this type of collective victimization, which include the situating of traumatic mental representations and unresolved psychological tasks into the psyches of subsequent generations. He then describes the process by which massive, shared trauma is continued through the generations and becomes a part of a large group's identity. This is a very rich and ambitious chapter which concludes with the author hoping that large group psychology becomes involved in interdisciplinary initiatives, provides information on large group identity and related concepts, and can be used by diplomats and other authorities in perpetuating the psychological well-being of large groups.

Prior to the conclusion, there are five chapters in the final section, which is titled "Psychoanalytic scholarship and activism." Robert Jay Lifton is one of the first people trained as a psychoanalyst to develop a psychoanalytically informed research methodology outside the office. Beginning his pioneering work in the 1950s, his studies have spanned the globe and encompassed different forms of mass violence over the last century. Interviewing people who had been subjected to Chinese thought reform or brainwashing, Hiroshima survivors, Vietnam vets, and even Nazi doctors, Lifton has contributed to our understanding of individual and group psychology in extreme circumstances and the historical basis for mass violence. He creatively combines psychoanalytic thought with the perspective of a historian.

For purposes of this book, we (Alpert and Goren) interviewed Dr. Lifton. Our interview focused on his being a psychoanalyst and doing the type of professional work that he does and on what theoretical and technical issues he thinks analysts might consider in being involved in social activism. He emphasizes his paradoxical relationship to psychoanalysis, making the point that everything he had done in his research depends on the existence of psychoanalysis that he found, when he began the work in the 1950s, to be inflexible and unyielding in theory and practice.

He considers what motivated him to do what he did, discusses his ideas about human nature, healing of individuals and communities, and reflects on his most painful professional experiences. In addition, he gives advice to psychoanalysts who are interested in working outside the consulting room. We are delighted to include parts of this interview in this volume. To our knowledge, there is considerable material included here that has not appeared in print before.

Next, this section includes the chapters by Mary-Joan Gerson, Nancy Hollander, and Elizabeth Hegeman. Each chapter, while quite different, attests to the myriad ways psychoanalysts can contribute to the application of psychoanalysis to the wider world and to social activism. Gerson describes her experience as a Fulbright Specialist in Namibia in 2012, seen through the lenses of her psychoanalytic perspective and of her previous experience in the Peace Corps in the 1960s. She concludes: "I was rerouted and redirected much of the time I taught and talked in Namibia but I rarely felt destabilized. My psychoanalytic training in self-reflection, privileging exploration, and tolerating uncertainty stood me well."

While Gerson writes about the work she did later in her career, Hollander writes about her activism work which preceded analytic training. Hollander acknowledges the profound influence of one of the founding mothers of analytic activism, Marie Langer. The latter had a major impact on the field and on Hollander's own work as an activist in Argentina and Nicaragua in extreme social situations of dictatorship and revolution, leading her eventually to become a psychoanalyst.

In yet another very different chapter, Hegeman applies psychoanalytic thinking to the situation involving the American Psychological Association and the role of psychologists in torture and interrogation at Guantanamo and illegal detention sites. She concludes that any effective review of ethical problems must consider the unconscious, institutional betrayal, motivations and insights, and the social, organizational, and structural barriers to ethics enforcement.

Bookending this section, Lewis Aron, in his chapter, reflects on Alpert's and Goren's interview with Robert Jay Lifton. He highlights some aspects of the psych-history of psychoanalysis regarding scholarship and activism, the micro and the macro, the individual and the socio-political, the scholar–clinician and the "psychoanalyst citizen." Aron, the director of NYU's Postdoctoral Program in Psychotherapy and Psychoanalysis, raises the issue of what psychoanalytic training programs must do in order to not lose potential candidates such as Dr. Lifton, who have so much to offer the field and the world. Aron concludes that, for purposes of the survival of psychoanalysis, we need a focus on the application of psychoanalysis to the wider world, to social activism, and to diversity.

In the final entry to this book, Alison Lake, Elizabeth R. Goren, and Judith L. Alpert provide a brief commentary on these chapters, with a particular focus on trauma and on the non-traditional, trauma-focused interventions our diverse contributors have proposed. The second part of this concluding chapter expands upon Aron's proposals for the future of psychoanalytic education.

In summary, we believe there are many reasons why we need to think about expanding our analytic identity. First, and most significant, we have something important to offer in these complex times, with so many national and international events and chronic conditions directly impacting the lives of Americans and around which psychoanalysts have been involved. Second, we can help the public have a better understanding of what psychoanalysis has to offer. Misconceptions abound about what we do and how we do it. Working in the community provides an opportunity for us to help, for our expertise to be known, and for us to communicate that there is an interiority underlying all human phenomena, a story underlying our individual and cultural histories.

References

Albee, G. W. (1970). The uncertain future of clinical psychology. *American Psychologist, 25*(12), pp. 1071–1080.

Altman, N. (2010). *The analysis in the inner city: Race, class and culture through a psychoanalytic lens*. Second Edition. New York: Routledge.

American Psychoanalytic Association. Committee for the Study of Social Issues. (1951). The dilemma of the analyst in a troubled world: A reply. *Bulletin of the American Psychoanalytic Association, 7*, pp. 70–72.

Aron, L. (1991). The patient's experience of the analyst's subjectivity. *Psychoanalytic Dialogues, 1*(1), pp. 29–51.

Aron, L. (2012). Psychoanalysis in the workplace: an introduction. *Psychoanalytic Dialogues, 22*(5), pp. 511–516.

Aron, L. & Starr, K. (2013). *A psychotherapy to the people: Toward a progressive psychoanalysis.* New York: Routledge.

Bernard, V. & Kelly, K. (1998). Some applications of psychiatry and psychoanalysis to social issues. *Psychoanalytic Review, 85*(1), pp. 139–170.

Bion, W. R. (1977). *Seven Servants*. New York: Jason Aronson Inc.

Canham, H. (2001). Exporting the Tavistock model to social services: Clinical consultative and teaching aspects. *Journal of Applied Psychoanalytic Studies, 3*(1), pp. 33–44.

Caplan, G. (1961). *An approach to community mental health.* London: Tavistock Publications.

Cushman, P. (1994).Confronting Sullivan's spider: Hermeneutics and politics of therapy. *Contemporary Psychoanalysis, 30*(4), pp. 800–844.

Cutler, D. L., Bevilacqua, J. & McFarland, B. H. (2003). Four decades of community mental health: A symphony in four movements. *Community Mental Health Journal, 39*(5), pp. 381–398.

Danto, E. (2005). *Freud's free clinics: Psychoanalysis & social justice, 1918–1938*. New York: Columbia University Press.

Dimen, M. (2011). With culture in mind: The social third introduction: Writing the clinical and the social. *Studies in Gender and Sexuality, 12*(1), 1–3.

Drake, R. E., Green, A. I., Mueser, K. T. & Goldman, H. H. (2003). The history of community mental health treatment and rehabilitation for persons with severe mental illness. *Community Mental Health Journal, 39*(5), pp. 427–440.

Erikson, E. (1950). *Childhood and society*. New York: Norton.

Felix, A. D. & Wine, P. R. (2001). From the couch to the street: Applications of psychoanalysis to work with individuals who are homeless and mentally ill. *Journal of Applied Psychoaanlaytic Studies*, *3*(1), pp. 17–32.

Freud, A. (1971). *The writings of Anna Freud. Volume VII Problems of psychoanalytic training, diagnosis, and the technique of therapy.* New York: International Universities Press.

Freud, S. (1933). Explanations, applications and orientations. In Strachey, J. (Ed.) *The Standard edition of the complete psychological works of Sigmund Freud*, Volume XX11 (1932–1936): New introductory lectures on psycho-analysis and other works. (pp. 136–157). London: The Hogarth Press and Institute of Psycho-analysis.

Fromm, E. (1955/1990). *The sane society.* New York: Owl Books.

Fromm, E. (1970). The crisis of psychoanalysis. In *The crisis of psychoanalysis: Essays on Freud, Marx and social psychology.* Greenwich: Fawcett Publications.

Goren, E. (2011). *Beyond the reach of ladders.* London: Open Gate Press.

Gourguechon, P. (2011). The citizen psychoanalyst: Psychoanalysis, social commentary, and social advocacy. *Journal of the American Psychoanalytic Association*, *59*(3), pp. 445–470.

Harris, A. (2005). *Gender as soft assembly.* New York: Routledge.

Horney, K. (1937/1999). *The neurotic personality of our time.* New York: Routledge.

Kernberg, O. (1976). *Object relations theory and clinical psychoanalysis.* New York: Aronson.

Kogan, I. (2004). The role of the analyst in the analytic cure during times of chronic crises. *Journal of the American Psychoanalytic Association*, *52*(3), pp. 735–757.

Kubie, L. (1950). The dilemma of the analyst in a troubled world. *Bulletin of the American Psychoanalytic Association*, *6*(4), pp. 1–4.

Layton, L. (2011). On the irreconcilable in psychic life: The role of culture in the drive to become both sexes. *Psychoanalytic Quarterly*, *8*(2), pp. 460–474.

Menzies, I. E. P. (1960). A case-study in the functioning of social systems as a defence against anxiety: a report on a study of the nursing service of a general hospital. *Human Relations*, *13*(2), pp. 95–121.

Mukherjee, P. P. & Alpert, J. L. (2006). Overview of psychological interventions in the acute aftermath of disaster. In L. Barbanel and R. J. Sternberg (Eds) *Psychological Interventions in Times of Crisis.* New York: Springer.

Oliner, S. (1996). External reality: The elusive dimension of psychoanalysis. *Psychoanalytic Quarterly*, *65*(2), pp. 267–300.

Philips, A. (1988). *Winnicott.* London: Fontana Paperbacks.

Sandler, P. & Alpert, J. (2000). Violence and group dynamics in the high school: The Columbine school shootings. *Journal for the Psychoanalysis of Culture and Society*, *5*(2), pp. 246–255.

Sarason, S. B. (1995). *Psychoanalysis, General Custer, and the verdicts of history and other essays on psychology on the social scene.* San Francisco: Jossey-Bass Publishers.

Sarason, S. B., Levine, M., Goldenberg, I., Cherlin, D. L. & Bennett, E. M. (1966). *Psychology in community settings: clinical, educational, vocational, social aspects.* New York: John Wiley & Sons.

Schmideberg, M. (1942). Some observations on individual reactions to air raids. *International Journal of Psycho-Analysis, 23*, pp. 146–176.

Sklarew, B., Twemlow, S. & Wilkinson, S. (2004). *Analysts in the trenches: Streets, schools, war zones*. Hillsdale: The Analytic Press.

Stein, M. (2004). The critical period of disasters: Insights from sense-making and psychoanalytic theory. *Human Relations, 57*(10), pp. 1243–1261.

Sullivan, H. S. (1948/2011). Towards a psychiatry of peoples. *Journal of Psychotherapy Integration, 21*(2), pp. 193–210.

Sullivan, H. S. (1955/2001). *The interpersonal theory of psychiatry.* New York: Routledge.

Sullivan, H. S. (2012). Conceptions of modern psychiatry: The First William Alanson White Memorial Lectures. *Psychiatry: Interpersonal and Biological Processes, 75*(1), pp. 3–17.

Twemlow, S. (2004). Psychoanalytic understanding of terrorism and massive social trauma. *Journal of the American Psychoanalytic Association, 52*(3), pp. 709–716.

Twemlow, S. & Parens, H. (2006). Might Freud's legacy lie beyond the couch? *Psychoanalytic Psychology, 23*(2), pp. 430–451.

Volkan, V. D. (1999a). Psychoanalysis and diplomacy, part I: Individual and large-group identity. *Journal of Applied Psychoanalytic Studies, 1*(2), pp. 29–55.

Volkan, V. D. (1999b). Psychoanalysis and diplomacy, part II: Large-group rituals. *Journal of Applied Psychoanalytic Studies, 1*(3), pp. 223–247.

Volkan, V. D. (1999c). The tree model: A comprehensive psychopolitical approach to unofficial diplomacy and the reduction of ethnic tension. *Mind and Human Interaction, 10*(3), pp. 142–210.

Westen, D. (2007). *The political brain: The role of emotion in deciding the fate of the nation.* New York: Public Affairs.

Winnicott, D. W. (1965/1990). *The maturational processes and the facilitating environment: Studies in the theory of emotional development.* First Reprint. London: Karnac Books.

Part I

Receiving testimony

Chapter 1

Reestablishing the internal "Thou" in testimony of trauma[1]

Dori Laub

Introduction

The following chapter highlights the therapeutic aspects of the testimonial intervention—an intervention that is also used in oral history and in the judicial context. Specifically, we are dealing here with the video testimonies of severely traumatized Holocaust survivors.

In two out of the three interview excerpts cited in this chapter, I served as the interviewer–listener. I was trying to promote a dialogic process between the survivor and myself and between the survivor and herself, in which her most severe traumatic experiences, perhaps for the first time in her life, were put into words. This chapter will repeatedly return to the special attributes of the dialogic process of trauma testimony.

The nature of traumatic experience

Philosophers, psychologists, psychiatrists, neuroscientists and writers have tried to convey the essence of massive psychic trauma. According to psychoanalyst Boulanger (2005), trauma "collapses" the distinction between the external world and internal experience: "when the external world becomes a direct reflection of our most terrifying thoughts, feelings, fantasies and nightmares, reality testing is irrelevant" (pp. 21–31). Cognitive functions, such as the reflective registration of external events and the observation of one's own responses to them, cease to operate under conditions of severe trauma. Tarantelli (2003) likens catastrophic psychic trauma to an explosion:

> In so far as an explosion disintegrates whatever is in its epicenter, it cannot be perceived or experienced or thought for there is nothing

> left to do so. Another way of saying this is that there is an utter absence, a radical break in being, an instant in which nothing exists (p. 915).

Jean Amery (1980), himself a survivor of the Gestapo torture chambers and of Auschwitz, writes:

> [B]ut only in torture does the transformation of the person into flesh become complete … The tortured person is only a body and nothing else besides that … The pain was what it was, beyond that there is nothing to say … [It marks] the limit of language to communicate (p. 33).

All three writers indicate that it is the *absence* of mental experience that characterizes massive psychic trauma because the mind is unable to register, cognitively and emotionally, the traumatic events. The self, as the interpreter of the experience and the creator of meaning, thus ceases to function.

On the nature of traumatic memories

According to Golden (2009), "The traumatic wound … excludes linguistic representation" (p. 82). "[It] outstrips discursive and representational resources" (Golden, 2009, p. 5). Yet traumatized people report so-called traumatic memories. These memories are indelible, sensory, affective, imprinted fragments that lack narrative cohesion and agency. These imprints of visual, auditory, olfactory, kinesthetic and physical sensations and strong affect remain outside a narrative structure, outside a story, even outside experience as it is remembered.

They are not subject to assimilation or to evolutionary change through integration into the associative network. They remain discrete, retaining their magnetic power in their contradictory, detailed and persistent clarity and also in the concomitant dense, yet absorbing, opaqueness that enshrouds them. They are qualitatively different from ordinary memories because they can continue to exert an influence on unconscious cognitive and emotional processes many years after the original traumatic event.

Memories of extreme traumatization: theoretical considerations

I would like now to propose a phenomenological formulation of traumatic memory emanating from what is called in psychoanalysis "object relations theory." Holocaust trauma—and genocide trauma for that matter—refuses knowledge because at its very core lies the complete failure of the empathic human dyad. The executioner does not heed the victim's plea for life; instead, he relentlessly proceeds with the execution. Human responsiveness came to be nonexistent in the death camps. A "Thou" responsive to one's basic needs no longer existed. Faith in the possibility of communication died; intrapsychically there was no longer a matrix of two people, a self and a resonating other. This despair of being able to communicate with others diminished the victims' ability to be in contact and in tune with themselves and to be able to register their own experience or reflect upon it.

Given that survivors of extreme traumatization experience a profound state of inner lonesomeness, it is necessary to explore the link between this traumatic state of loneliness—of objectlessness—and the absence of communicable thought. For traumatic sensation to be experienced as thought, it must undergo the process of symbolization. According to Melanie Klein (1930), it is "not only [that] symbolism [comes] to be the foundation of all fantasy and sublimation, but more than that, it is the basis of the subject's relation to the outside world and to reality, in general" (p. 221). Therefore, to perceive, recognize or participate in reality, the process of symbolization needs to be in place. "Symbol formation," according to Hannah Segal (1991), "governs the capacity to communicate, since all communication is made by means of symbols" (p. 395). She proceeds, "Symbols are needed in not only communication with the external world, but also in internal communication," that is, with oneself (Segal, 1991, p. 395). "The capacity to communicate with oneself by using symbols is, I think, the basis of verbal thinking, which is the capacity to communicate with oneself by means of words" (Segal, 1991, p. 396). When the empathic other totally fails in the external world of the death camps, the internal, empathic "Thou," the means for self-dialogue, ceases to exist. The ongoing internal dialogue, the internal "I" speaking to the internal "Thou," which allows for historicity, narrative and meaning to unfold, falls silent. Sensory impressions, no matter how powerful, remain fragments that do not coalesce. Thus, the two-part sequence consisting first, of the destruction of the internal "other" object and, second, of the failure of the process of symbolization through internal dialogue, leads to the absence of conscious experience and also to the absence of repressed memory. It is as though memory in its wider form becomes nonexistent, a state which very much fits with Van der Kolk, McFarlane and Weisaeth's description (1996) of traumatic memories as the return of "emotional and sensory states with little capacity for verbal representation" (p. 296).

The above-described processes that promote the shutdown of the mental registering processes, the cessation of the dialogue with the internal "Thou" (and, ultimately, of symbolization and thought), lead to a certain absence, or rather erasure, of memory. Primo Levi (cited in Tarantelli, 2003) poignantly described this phenomenon in his account of the *Musselmänner* state that he witnessed in the death camps. The "absence of any 'trace of thought'" (Levi, 1987, p. 96) "... [pointed to] a destruction of all mental activity that had a full individuality, subjectivity, or personal being" (Tarantelli, 2003, p. 917). Hence, the narration of this state from within becomes impossible.

Testimony as a relibidinization of the fragments

Testimony is a powerful, libido-driven process of putting fragments together, creating a whole, making such a whole a part of one's experiential landscape in a temporal, historical sequence, historicizing it, restoring the narrative flow and associatively linking it to other experiences and to the experiencing "I." Testimony is a process of symbolizing the concrete so that the traumatic experience can become communicable to oneself and known and transmittable to an "other," thus producing an experience that can be known, remembered, transmitted and forgotten.

According to psychoanalytic theory, an object is passionately yearned for and desperately needed to make this libidinally charged testimonial process possible. This object is the addressee, an intimate companion for the journey into yet-uncharted territory—a totally present, listening "Thou." Such a listening "Thou" is the *sine qua non*, the indispensable condition for the dialogic process between the internal "I" and the internal "Thou" to resume.

Let us turn now to the video testimony itself. To begin, the witness identifies herself by stating her name and the date and place of her birth. She is then invited to delve into early family and childhood memories. Personal experience and images are emphasized. The interviewer asks her to imagine sitting at a living-room table and opening an album of old faded photos; he asks her to describe what she sees. She is invited to view her own self-made movie that starts rolling in her mind and to relate what she sees. What she relates is immediate, personal and visual. The interviewer allows his own imagination to flow as he takes in the visual, the auditory and the kinesthetic, all that is transmitted in the testimony. The fine nuances in the tone of voice, body movement and posture and facial expression—all of these are very important for the interviewer to take in. The interviewer's own flow of associations complements the multimodal transmittals in the testimony and informs his interventions.

Finding the "Thou" in the testimonial relationship

Witnesses and listeners have a common goal—jointly to visit a lived experience of extremity, to step into the place in which neither of them had been before. Literally speaking, the witness has been there, but experientially she had been absent from it. Caruth's concept (1996) of the "unclaimed experience" is very helpful here. At the moment the trauma occurred, the person who was affected was not there to experience it. She is quite aware of her absence, of having missed it, and feels compelled to return to it and at the same time terrified to come near it. As pointed out earlier, it is a place of utter aloneness. Therefore, the promise of a companion–listener who will join her makes such a venture thinkable, perhaps even inviting; the hope is that she will experience a henceforth foreclosed moment of intense intimacy.

The companion–listener echoes such feelings of anticipation, being aware at the same time of the responsibility she is taking on—not to flinch at whatever she hears or experiences, and to let nothing detract from her total presence in, and to, the moment. Her goal is to facilitate what the witness anticipates, which is an encounter with herself, a homecoming to a most profound personal truth, a foray into a territory she had either fearfully and carefully avoided or allowed herself to experience only on a separate, parallel track, as though it belonged to someone else.

In order to integrate the traumatic fragments and turn them into real knowledge, the survivor needs to locate the fervently yearned-for dialogic "Thou" within herself. She can do so by finding a trustworthy, passionate and totally present companion–listener in whom she can temporarily anchor that internal "Thou." That listener has not only to be totally present, but also ahead of the survivor in the place of trauma, patiently waiting for her there. She has to assist her actively by providing a holding frame of time, space and sequence, and she must actively intervene when the survivor is overwhelmed by her feelings, at a loss for words and faltering because she cannot sustain the effort or wants to flee the terror, grief and pain.

It is this form of passionately involved, active listening that the interviewer offers to the survivor through the process of the video testimony. The listening sets in motion the "coming together" of the disjointed traumatic fragments into a hitherto unknown, cohesive narrative, which often surprises the survivor herself. By hearing herself she realizes that, at the outset, she had not known all that she knew. Undoubtedly, other audiences besides the current companion–listener—past, present and future audiences—are implicitly, although most likely unconsciously, addressed in the video testimony, whereby it becomes a historical event in itself. It is through the restoration of her internal "Thou" that the survivor is able to tell the story of her experience—both to herself and to society at large.

Testimony and psychoanalysis

Testimony is a meeting place for the witnessing and repair of trauma-induced fragmented memories and psychic disruption. The testimonial intervention responds to, and addresses, that which has been deeply wounded and not found an opportunity to heal in the trauma survivor. A psychoanalytic understanding of the interviewer and interviewee relationship during the testimonial intervention not only vastly contributes to our understanding of the traumatic damage but also informs us about the healing processes that need to be set in motion to repair it.

The uniqueness of the testimonial intervention lies in the fact that there is always an event, an experience—although it may cover a lifetime—that is known to be there, even if it has hitherto not been consciously formulated. Thus it is information that has yet to be recorded and brought to an addressee—to a party interested in receiving it. Testimony is therefore an urgent transmittal of information. There is an unrelenting internal pressure to convey it, as well as an external readiness and eagerness to receive it.

When such transmittal has been accomplished, the survivor no longer is, or feels, alone with the inexpressible extreme experience. She is less helplessly prey to its devastating impact. The internal cauldron of sensations and affects has been put into the frame of a sequential narrative; it can now be remembered, transmitted and forgotten. However, such narrative is never complete, and highly charged blank spots of the inexpressible (almost unimaginable) experience persist, exerting their magnetic power on the survivor, who feels compelled endlessly to revisit them while at the same time constantly fleeing their proximity.

These intense, affect-laden voids of memory—which, to begin with, can obliterate the traumatic experience in its entirety—constitute the power source that drives testimony and exerts the pressure for its deliverance. This mechanism holds true for a broad range of experiences of extreme trauma. In personal observations, I have found that cancer survivors, when feeling safe in the company of other survivors, are similarly driven to "tell their story" of their encounters with death. A group of chronically hospitalized "psychotic" Holocaust survivors, interviewed in Israel in recent years, experienced the same internal pressure to bear witness (Laub, 2005; Strous et al., 2005; Kaplan and Laub, 2009). Unfortunately, their capacity to symbolize, free associate, reflect and verbalize has been so profoundly damaged by the chronicity of their condition (lasting for decades), their social isolation and their somatic treatments (insulin shock, ECT and psychotropic medication), that all they were able to create was a constricted, static and fragmented narrative.

The goal of traditional psychoanalysis, on the other hand, is to allow for the emergence of the unconscious through the method of free association and the elucidation of the transference experience. There is no particular force, no inner compulsion that drives an analysis, no story that reaches for words. Rather, it is characterized by surrender to the wanderings of the mind, enabled by the feeling that one is protected by the analyst's nonjudgmental presence and neutrality. It has a rhythm set by the frequency of the sessions, and it lacks an endpoint in time. Dreams, parapraxes, transference experiences and enactments and, last but not least, remembrances provide the scaffolding along which the analytic narrative unfolds. Although there is no explicit addressee in traditional analysis, the analyst's emotional presence implicitly fulfills that function and becomes the equivalent of the testimonial "Thou."

Indeed, psychoanalytic literature is replete with references to the internal good object, a concept that usually highlights the infant's relationship with the mother. Freud's (1930, 1961, p. 11) concept of the "oceanic feeling"—being one with the universe—that arises from the oneness with the mother in the womb, Margaret Mahler's (1967) concept of the developmental phase of symbiosis, Winnicott's (1953) "transitional space," Henry Parens' (1970) "inner sustainment," Mahler et al.'s (1975) "object constancy" and Kohut's (1971) "self object"—all of these concepts address processes that are essential for internal representation and symbolization to occur. And it is these processes that constitute core components of the testimonial intervention.

Within the spectrum of psychoanalytically informed therapeutic interventions, the testimonial process possesses three unique elements: the internal pressure to transmit and tell; the real story that is "there"; and the yearning for, and presence of, a listener who receives it. On close scrutiny, these three elements do not place testimony in a category that is separate from psychoanalysis. Both processes—testimony and psychoanalysis—are in essence dialogic. The analysand does not speak to a void, even if he speaks to himself. In such a case, it is his own internal good object, projected onto the analyst, which he addresses. In both testimony and psychoanalysis, the narrative deepens and branches out, taking turns that may come as a surprise to the narrator. Freud's dictum, "where id was, ego shall be" (1933, 1964, p. 80) applies to both, although in the lengthier psychoanalysis this transformation can go much further than in the single session testimony. Furthermore, a process is set in motion in both, a process that can continue on its own, far beyond the time frame of the psychoanalytic or the testimonial event. This process includes, but is not limited to, symbolization, self-reflection and remembering. While it is not a particular event that serves as an organizing principle as in the case of testimony, psychoanalysis too leads to the recovery of memories that may emerge as organizing principles and potential building blocks of the psychoanalytic narrative. What remains, the basic difference between testimony and traditional psychoanalysis, may be limited to the inner intense pressure to transmit and the experience of transmittal itself, which are at the center of the testimonial intervention. The latter can, therefore, be seen as a piece of psychoanalytic work that is limited in scope and that does not include parapraxes, transference or dream work.

The testimonial momentum may also be operative in traditional psychoanalysis, when traumatic experience is involved. At such a juncture, it becomes the process that fuels the therapeutic action and provides the impetus for clinical movement and flow. It would be methodologically very difficult to isolate and study it in the context of a traditional psychoanalysis; therefore, the nontraditional modality of the testimonial intervention provides the most suitable research setting for capturing and investigating in depth the testimonial momentum.

Testimonial examples

I shall now present three brief excerpts of video testimonies of different survivors; in each case, I believe the internal "Thou" is absent or present to different degrees. I shall discuss each excerpt in detail in terms of the absence or presence of that internal addressee.

Interview with Helen K. (1985)

SURVIVOR: My mother was taken a few days before and then they took us all to Majdanek.

INTERVIEWER: Your husband too?

SURVIVOR: My husband too, myself. But, so … when we went to Majdanek it was just the most terrible. As much as I experienced bad things after, but this was … they put us in cattle cars. They pushed in I don't know how many people, but they really wanted us to die. And, we were on those wagons, uh … I don't know how many people were there, but my brother died in my arms. My younger brother was [pause] hahh, and my husband's two sisters. There was not enough oxygen for all those people and they kept us in those wagons for days. They wanted us to die in the wagons. You know the cattle cars with very little windows [pause], hhhaa.

INTERVIEWER: How old was your brother?

SURVIVOR: Maybe thirteen, he wasn't even Bar Mitzvahed. You know when my brother died in my arms, I said to myself, I'm going to live, I must be the only survivor from my family. I'm going to live. I made up my mind that I'm going to defy Hitler. I'm not going to give in, because he wants me to die, so I'm going to live. I am just going to be very, very strong.

Comments on Helen K.

It is as though this woman, Helen K., who had lived in the Warsaw Ghetto, in Mila 18—the very building from which the Jewish uprising was staged and had herself witnessed the uprising, its defeat and the brutal reprisal that followed—only at the moment when her brother asphyxiated in her arms, became fully cognizant of the Nazi murderous intent against her. It is as though a paradigm shift had occurred; the internal "Thou" was represented and she finally became aware of the intended destruction that awaited her.

Helen K. rises to the challenge and refuses to submit. Her inner dialogue—"I said to myself I'm going to live. I must be the only survivor from my family. I am going to live. I made up my mind that I am going to defy Hitler"—is Helen K.'s confrontation with the "Thou." It is possible that the immensity of the pain of having so abruptly lost her brother resuscitated an image of her internal "Thou" with whom she could regain connection and have a dialogue that enabled the intent and strategy to defy Hitler. The acute grief and rage at the shocking death of her younger brother do not lead her to identify with the victim, but crystallize in her a sense of identity, significance and agency, as well as a recognition of the mortal enemy she wants to defeat.

Interview with Bessie K. (1985)

SURVIVOR: They took us with the bus to an airfield and nearby were trains, the cattle trains. And um, as I look back … I think for a while I was in a daze. I didn't know what was happening actually. I saw them taking away the men separate, the children separate, and the women separate. So I had a baby. I took the coats that I had, the bundles and I wrapped them around the baby. And I put it, I put it on the left side. Because I saw that the Germans were saying left to right. And I went through with the baby, but the baby was short of breath, so it started to choke and it started to cry. So the German called me back and he says, "What do you have there?" in German.

SURVIVOR: Now, I didn't know what to do, everything was so fast, happened so suddenly. I wasn't prepared for it. To look back, the experience … I think I was numb or something happened to me. I don't know. I wasn't there even. And um, he stretched out his arms, I should hand him over the bundle. I hand him over the bundle and this was the last time I had the bundle.

SURVIVOR: When I look back, I don't think I had anybody with me. I was alone. I was within myself. Since that time, I think all my life I've been alone, even when I met Jack. I didn't tell Jack my past. Jack just found out recently. I think to me, I was dead. I died and I didn't want to hear nothing, I didn't want to know nothing, and I didn't want to talk about it and I didn't want to admit to myself that this happened to me.

SURVIVOR: In Stuttgart I found the doctor who operated on me, in the Ghetto. And they brought us in there and when she saw me there, she was so happy to see me. Right away she said to me, "Where's the baby? What happened to the baby?" And right there, I said, "What baby?" I said to the doctor, "What baby?" I didn't have a baby. I don't know of any baby. That is what it did to me.

Comments on Bessie K.

What is striking are Bessie K.'s own observations on her state of utter, stark "aloneness" during her experience of losing her baby and throughout the rest of her life. She remarks on several occasions that she didn't have anyone and she was alone. There is no "Thou," no internal or external "other" with whom she can experience a resonance, an echo of what she has gone through.

Earlier in the interview she spoke of having given birth to a baby in Ghetto Kovno, where pregnancies and the delivery of babies were strictly forbidden and punishable by death. She spoke of finding food for the baby and building him a rocking chair. Even during the selection, the baby was still present to her; she goes through with the baby. But the baby was short of breath and started to choke and cry. And the German called her back and asked her, in German, what she had there. From then onwards, there was no longer a baby, no longer a child.

At that moment in her testimony, the bundle took the place of the "other" and the pantomime of the bundle began. Its three steps were: (a) He stretched out his arms. I should hand him over the bundle; (b) I hand him over the bundle; (c) This was the last time I had the bundle.

There is only silence—no voice. No inner dialogue takes place. The inner "Thou" is no more. Her response to the doctor's inquiry about the baby is "What baby? … I don't know of any baby." The testimony, as it unfolds, shows the failure to symbolize, relate, represent and remember—it is compellingly clear. It all ceased with the murder of one baby.

Interview with Leon W. (2005) describing his return to his hometown, Lodz, shortly after the end of the war in the hope of finding family members alive

LEON: I came over into the house, nobody there. If I, I remember opening the door to our big one-room apartment and …

INTERVIEWER: And nobody there … it's terrible. That was a big blow.

LEON: Enough [silence, tearing, trying to speak].

INTERVIEWER: And you left? Lodz.

LEON: That's right [crying], yes.

INTERVIEWER: I assumed that you realized that if you …

LEON: That is my worst …

INTERVIEWER: Yes [pause]. Until that time there was still hope, I understand. [silence, tearing]

LEON: Ahh, I think that was my … when I came into the house, in the room this is …

INTERVIEWER: Ahem.

LEON: That was … that is …

INTERVIEWER: Is?

LEON: It was seriously, at that time it dawned on me, what happened. Not through all the years, only until that time. I walked into the house and I looked at that empty room. It was a house, a house, just one room. And I noticed … what do you call it? A little bulge over there, so my parents must have put a couple of items there, pictures. And that is how I have some pictures from the Ghetto, from my sisters. That is the … every time I think of, it is the highlight of my … [pause] oh my god, it's 2:30 already.

INTERVIEWER: Does this moment …

LEON: Yeah …

INTERVIEWER: This moment keep coming back?

LEON: Yeah, it will come back. Yeah, but I … I … but not when I was young, just the last few years.

Comments on Leon W.

Leon is reliving his fantasy, hopeful in the expectation of finding, even meeting somebody from his family there in the big room. Instead he found "nobody there." The encounter is with the empty room, with the gaping absence, the nearly overwhelming pain and grief he feels entering the room, in which he does not find the parents and sibling he had hoped would be there. As long as he had not yet entered the empty room, he still believed it would not be empty, although intellectually he knew better. Only now does it dawn on him what happened. His family is very present, though, through the pain of its absence.

He struggles with his pain through his crying and wiping off his tears, his inability to speak, through wanting to stop ("Enough"), through communicating that this was his "worst," and, most of all, through his hesitance to enter the empty room. It is only at his fourth attempt, after conceding that it was "at that time it dawned on me what happened," that he is able to relate the rest of the story: walking into the house and looking at that empty room, and noticing the bulge—where his parents must have left a message, putting a couple of pictures, for him. In this way he imaginatively meets them again, while once more confronted with the pain of their absence. It is noteworthy that Leon does not give up confronting his pain, even when I offer him the opportunity to speak about leaving the town of Lodz. He is fully engaged in addressing it and himself through his utterances and his self-reflections. There is definitely an internal "Thou" present, although he may be momentarily choked up with tears. I notice my repeated attempts to lighten his struggle by putting into words what I think he cannot say. However, I think it was my persevering presence, more than the content of what I said, that may have helped him resolve the crisis of witnessing that he had gone through.

This excerpt contains a series of encounters—with nobody, with himself (that was his worst, that is when it dawned on him what happened), with his parents' message (pictures), with the moment that keeps coming back, and perhaps with me.

The therapeutic action of testimony

Testimony is the return to the personal experience of a severely traumatizing historical event (or any severely traumatizing external event) that opens the possibility for an alternative, different psychological outcome. Historical fact cannot be changed. The dead cannot be brought back to life; the home that was lost cannot be found; the injury that was inflicted cannot be undone. What was destroyed may remain in ruins; the boundaries that were so violently breached may never be intact again. The horror that was made real may last forever; yet the process described by Jean Amery's (1980) statement may be reversed through the process of testimony: "The expectation of help, the certainty of help, is indeed one of the fundamental experiences of human beings … But with the first blow … against which there can be no defense and which no helping hand will ward off... *[one] can no longer feel at home in the world*" (pp. 28–29, p. 40).

Trauma, when relived and reexperienced in the context of dialogue with an empathic listener, may restore, to a degree, the victim's sense of being at home in the world. There is no longer the utter aloneness and incommunicability that is part of the extreme traumatic experience. Once such dialogue (mostly with the internal "Thou") is reestablished, traumatic narrative can unfold and be transmitted. Once narrativized and transmitted, the indigestible fragments of traumatic sensations and affect occupy less space and exert less pressure on, and in, the emotional life of the survivor. Thus, psychologically, history can be repaired and what is broken can, to a degree, be mended.

Concluding remarks

Extreme trauma is a psychophysiological event. A wide spectrum of physiological and psychological theories attempts to elucidate its mechanisms. Recent neuroscience research data allow us to map the rough contours of the neuronal event—a stress hormone and a mediated short-circuiting of both the hippocampus (instrumental in converting short- into long-term memory and integrating experience into symbolic thought) and the prefrontal cortex. On the other end of the spectrum of research approaches, traditional psychoanalytic theory suggests that the breach of the stimulus barrier caused by excessive traumatic excitation leads to the disintegration of the self and of the registering psychic apparatus.

While both approaches offer a general understanding of the psychological phenomenology of extreme traumatic experience, neither specifically examines this phenomenology in order to glean from it a more precise understanding of its unique experiential dimension. Both stop short of looking at such experience from "the inside." From what we know about the processes of registration, retention and recall of extreme trauma, we can attempt to infer such an "inside story." There is no question that it begins with massive annihilation anxiety. The abrupt cessation of internal mental representation leads us to believe that such annihilation anxiety is secondary to the trauma-induced loss of the sustained internal good object with whom the experiencing "I" is in constant dialogue, and which enables us to symbolize and narrativize experience. Thus, traumatic perception does not become a narrativized experience and it remains fragmented, intense and held in abeyance. It is only when the desperate search and yearning for such a lost good object finds resonance in the passionate interest of a listening other, a witness to the witness in the process of testimony, that the mental representation of the good object, in the form of an internal "Thou," begins to reemerge, making a resumption of dialogic narrative flow possible. The experiencing "I," having rediscovered its internal counterpart, can narrativize and historicize the paralyzing trauma fragments, and so create a more coherent trauma narrative. Thus testimony has a therapeutic effect because it allows the survivor both to recover the memory of the past and to live more fully in the present.

Note

1 Reprinted from *Psychoanalysis, Culture & Society, suppl. Special Issue: Psychoanalysis, Trauma, and Community* 18.2 (Jun 2013): 184–198 by permission of Palgrave Macmillan.

References

Amery, J. (1980) *At the Mind's Limits: Contemplation by a Survivor on Auschwitz and its Realities*. Bloomington, IN: Indiana University Press.

Bessie, K. (1985) [Video recording of Bessie K] Holocaust Testimony. *Fortunoff Video Archive*. Yale University, New Haven, CT.

Boulanger, G. (2005) From voyeur to witness: Recapturing symbolic function after psychic trauma. *Psychoanalytic Psychology* 22: 21–31.

Caruth, C. (1996) *Unclaimed Experience: Trauma, Narrative and History*. Baltimore, MD: Johns Hopkins University Press.

Freud, S. (1930, 1961) Civilization and its discontents. *Standard Edition* 21. London, England: Hogarth Press, pp. 57–146.

Freud, S. (1933, 1964) New introductory lectures on psycho-analysis. *Standard Edition* 22. London, England: Hogarth Press, pp. 3–182.

Golden, K. (2009) Trauma and speech as an adaptation in Merleau-Ponty. In: K. Golden and B. Bergo (eds) *The Trauma Controversy: Philosophical and Interdisciplinary Dialogues*. Albany, NY: SUNY Press, pp. 5–8.

Helen, K. (1985) [Video recording of Helen K.] Holocaust Testimony. *Fortunoff Video Archive*. Yale University, New Haven, CT.

Kaplan, S. and Laub, D. (2009) Affect regulation in extreme traumatization-fragmented narratives of Holocaust survivors. *The Scandinavian Psychoanalytic Review* 32 (2): 93–104.

Klein, M. (1930) The importance of symbolic formation in the development of the ego. *International Journal of Psychoanalysis* 11: 24–39.

Kohut, H. (1971) *The Analysis of the Self.* New York, NY: International Universities Press.

Laub, D. (2005) From speechlessness to narrative: The cases of Holocaust historians and of psychiatrically hospitalized survivors. *Literature and Medicine* 24 (2): 253–265.

Leon, W. (2005) [Video recording of Leon W.] Forced Labor Testimony. *Forced Labor 1939–1945 Archive*. Free University of Berlin, Berlin, Germany.

Levi, P. (1987) *If This is A Man; The Truce*. London, England: Abacus.

Mahler, M. (1967) On human symbiosis and the vicissitudes of individuation. *Journal of the American Psychoanalytic Association* 15: 740–763.

Mahler, M., Pine, F. and Bergman, A. (1975) *The Psychological Birth of the Human Infant: Symbiosis and Individuation*. New York, NY: Basic Books.

Parens, H. (1970) Inner sustainment: Metapsychological considerations. *Psychoanalytic Quarterly* 39: 223–239.

Segal, H. (1991) *Dream, Phantasy and Art*. London, England: Tavistock/Routledge.

Strous, R.D., Weiss, M., Felsen, I., Finkel, B., Melamed, Y., Bleich, A., Kotler, M. and Laub, D. (2005) Video testimony of long-term hospitalized psychiatrically ill Holocaust survivors. *American Journal of Psychiatry* 162 (12): 2287–2294.

Tarantelli, C.B. (2003) Life within death: Towards a metapsychology of catastrophic psychic trauma. *The International Journal of Psychoanalysis* 84 (4): 915–928.

Van der Kolk, B.A., McFarlane, A.C. and Weisaeth, L. (1996) *Traumatic Stress: The Effects of Overwhelming Experience on Mind, Body and Society*. New York, NY: Guilford Press.

Winnicott, D.W. (1953) Transitional objects and transitional phenomena. *International Journal of Psychoanalysis* 34: 89–97.

Chapter 2

Dwelling at the thresholds[1]

Witnesses to historical trauma across concentric fields

Judy Roth

Overtime, I have had the privilege to listen to stories from people living in the Middle East and to consult to some projects. This work changed my voice as a psychoanalyst. Clinical questions emerged that became a hub for new inquiry and networking that revolved around the following questions: What kind of witnessing presence—what kind of "accompaniment"[2]—can psychoanalysts bring to a zone of continuous and sequential trauma (Keilson, 1992)? How can we amplify the real voices of people living at the edges of what we can grasp let alone engage without betraying the stories we have had the privilege to hold? That is, can we reach for psychological truths without objectifying, simplifying, appropriating, and further "othering" the very voices we seek to humanize? And might there be some way to create a responsive presence that would be preventative of later damage?

I was interested in the ripple effects of trauma and resilience as these radiated out from those most directly impacted to those less so, and I believed that if we heard voices from different points along the continuum, we would not only learn about the impact of this particular historical epoch but we would have a clearer sense of how to stand in solidarity with those living with dehumanization and oppression without igniting more circles of domination.

My interest in the question of how we bear and transform the reverberations of social trauma stemmed from work with young adults in the inner city, many of them immigrants wrestling with refugee legacies, and from my own coming to terms with the lives of my parents, Holocaust refugees. It was not an accident that my work gravitated to witnessing in Israel–Palestine. My mother had escaped to Palestine as a child, and later, when

I became a mother, I wrestled with what to teach myself and my children about realities in Israel. This struggle ignited the question of why it is so hard to see Palestinian anguish while bearing in mind Jewish pain.

I carry a conviction that while social trauma reverberates across generations, so can responsive witnessing, in ways that are not only game-changing but life-changing. It is a conviction that stems from knowing that many responsible bystanders stepped in to rescue my mother, who was a "hidden child." Additionally, my family has had the privilege of dialoguing with children and grandchildren of German bystanders and Nazi perpetrators from my father's village in Germany. These relationships not only validated pain and a shared history of evil, but also neutralized what I was primed to hate, making it possible to "legitimately" reckon with outrage and to imagine a way out.

Circles of witnessing

By definition, zones of continuous trauma, as in the ongoing political conflict in Israel and Palestine, are chaotic and overwhelming, ever-changing and yet, relentlessly the same. These are blazing and compelling relational minefields that are at once violently reactive, saturated with meaning and history, and choking with their own intensity. The atmosphere can be dramatic but also terrifyingly empty, as civility insidiously fractures, and these fractures are then disavowed. So where are the points of entry for the social witness? And what kind of presence can we bring? And how do we locate ourselves and know vis-a-vis who we are standing with and what ripples of social trauma we are each holding? Can our psychoanalytical understanding shed light on this complicated whirl of humanity and inform ways of accompanying those caught in its grip?

I want to envisage those implicated in the continuous traumas of political violence in Palestine and Israel—both near and far—in concentric circles,[3] in the hopes that visualizing this complicated field will make it easier to see and engage. So imagine concentric circles: At the center of these circles are children, the most vulnerable to the long-lasting impact of social traumas. Surrounding them are their parents and families and then educators and community and religious leaders. Finally, at the outer rims are humanitarian workers, caring professionals, the concerned local public, and then all of us, more remote and concerned others. These circles of stakeholders are holding ripples of the same traumatic contagions and wear several hats, as victims, bystanders, sometimes perpetrators, and always witnesses. They carry the psychic and collective accommodations to ongoing war—the longings for peace, reparation, and justice and the more primitive wish for revenge. But they also carry the wish to live, the strong traditions and tribal bonds, and the intense intimacy and passions.

If trauma is "suffering in excess of what the psyche can absorb" (Hoffman, 2004, p. 54), nesting social trauma within these fields of others is enormously helpful conceptually and clinically. It enables us to see how traumatic contagions of trauma vibrate across communities,[4] and it allows us to acknowledge the more silent voices impacted by social trauma. It also enables us to imagine that each ring of witnesses provides some containment for the others along the radius (Ad-Dab'bagh, 2015) and to think about how communities might maximize this possibility.

Nesting the voices also clarifies how we, as witnessing-outsiders, are embedded, helping us define our role and port of entry. While our engagements might include collecting testimonies, supervision, consultation, and project development, our mandate remains twofold: Developing a form of responsive witnessing that is, in the words of Leonard Grob (2016), "...a way of 'being with' those who survive atrocity and other evils, that is not about an 'accounting' for suffering, nor an overidentification with anguish that we can never hope to grasp." But rather, Grob is calling for an "attentiveness" to suffering, a "wakefulness" (a concept he extends from Levinas) that "troubles us with brutal clarity and leaves us with the pain that evil inflicts."

Implicit in this stance, is another mandate: To stand in a particular kind of "solidarity." This solidarity can be defined as opening a space (Long, personal communication)—a space in which we are invited to partner in amplifying that which is unacknowledged, to grasp what defies communication, and to be mindful of our privileged and limited access to the subjective impact of specific political realities (Ullman, 2011; Roth and Duaibis, 2015).

This chapter will use concentric circles as the metaphoric topography wide enough to contain the multiple realities of those living in this zone of continuous trauma. I will amplify stories from Israelis, Palestinians, and internationals standing at different places along these circles to illustrate how fields of others are wrestling with echoes of the same traumatic contagions. I will begin with the participants in a truth commission and move to Palestinian parents and children living in the more embattled friction zones, and then to the human rights workers and professionals who work with them. Collectively, their stories highlight what is at stake on this frontline.

Prelude: the crucible

In one of the first experiments with a truth commission in an ongoing conflict zone,[5] elderly Palestinian and Israeli Jewish men have been invited to publically tell their stories of displacement, expulsion, and conquest. The gathering, initiated by a human rights organization working to promote acknowledgment of Palestinian history and the ongoing injustices Palestinians have suffered, takes place in Southern Israel four months after the war in Gaza has ended (Operation Cast Lead, summer 2014), at a time when many Bedouin villages in the area are facing the threat of losing their land and villages.

It is a riveting and excruciating gathering where volunteer professionals and a small, salaried staff has come together to prepare these men, a commission, and a concerned public wanting to hear and learn. I had joined wanting to learn about testifying and witnessing in truth commissions. Later, I was asked to think about how to support those testifying at the public hearing.

In a climate where the existential questions of who is legitimate, who possesses, and who is dispossessed pulses through so many relational and systemic dynamics, the challenge was how to keep these men's voices primary, how to assure that the authorship and control of their stories remained theirs, and how to minimize the opening of wounds (see Hamber, 2009). Repeatedly, at the beginning of each man's presentation, participants are reminded that these men have a special place in the hall, that their stories are theirs, and that their courage enables a process to begin. The unstated pulsates: How far do you push elderly men to recall? What might explode in this ambiance of civility and stature? What are the objectives, since no justice can be rectified until the Israeli–Palestinian conflict is resolved? And can dignity be assured? And so, with complicated and modest hope that Israelis might establish a more human record of historical accuracy and might begin to bear witness to Palestinian pain and claims, a process unfolds.

It is clear that the men testifying are taking a risk: The accepted and lauded history of the majority of Israeli Jews inverts in this gathering, a counter-culture of sorts. The Jewish fighters move from being seen as the hero-fighters in their own communities, to perpetrators. As they begin to speak, they are now victims to an audience of internationals, Palestinians, and Israelis desperately wanting what is impossible—accountability and reparation. The Palestinians on the commission do the impossible: They must remain professional and formulate questions in a situation where their own families have either been historically and/or currently devastated. They want answers to the hardest questions of all: Were Jewish fighters aware that expulsions, looting, sexual assaults, and killing happened to communities of real human beings? Were they aware that lives fell apart, that the pain that ensued still bears down? This unique audience is challenged, in turn, with the task of trying to keep all players human, even those responsible for atrocities. They must contain feelings related to a history of losses—some recent and raw—which have never been fully acknowledged, if at all (see Even-Tzur, 2016).

An elderly, Jewish man, identified as a "Jewish fighter" begins to speak: "I came here to tell you about my participation in the War of Independence." He moves into his story composed, assuring the commission that he and his brigade were sent to fight Egyptians and not evacuate Palestinians. The commissioners, first calmly and then, with greater urgency probe, wanting him to know more than he says he knows. Does he feel badly for what happened in the past? For what is happening now? Does he think actions were justified?

When he is pressed but does not disclose any role in evacuating, expelling, or looting, nor knowledge of how Palestinians were prevented from returning, he frustrates and disappoints. He asserts that he and his brigade did nothing wrong, that Jews are caring and protective both then and now, "We saw this in the last operation (Gaza), not to harm." The room stirs, and the organizers ask for quiet. The commissioners ask one more question, even as this man tires: "Did he participate in exploding homes and was he aware of artillery bombardment?" Was he aware? That is the question that lingers and haunts. Was he aware that lives were impacted, individuals violated, and families devastated? Did he register the suffering, then and now? And does Palestinian suffering matter?

As this elderly man is questioned about his role in events, he flushes and coughs, as if he is losing not only public stature but becoming psychically stranded. Where are we? In the past, 1948, or the summer of 2014, or four months later? A worry ignites that this man does not look okay. "We are lynching him," a Palestinian later whispered, clearly worried and moved. Others in the room are angry as they hear him speak. What happens if we collectively bring this man to a place where he walks too far and fast through the looking glass, if too much comes alive? While extensively prepared for the presentation, no one could prepare him for what it would feel like to tell his story and have it questioned publically. And what about the Palestinians in the room who have grandparents or parents who were forced to flee, or displaced, or more recently have had family members who have been injured, killed, or subject to injustice? What does it take to sit calmly, as if the history of the past can be divorced from urgent realities of today and the familial and collective traumas they carry?

There is no escaping what Vamik Volkan (2001) so incisively describes as the activation of collective identifications, the "time collapse" that ensues when traumatic memories are triggered, or the entitlement to regain what was in flames. The commission's need to "get to the truth," which likely touched on the audience's as well, creates a force of its own, the Golem now out of the box. Kaethe Weingarten, drawing on Volkan's work, warns that in the face of "psychic energy longing to reverse ancestral humiliation" (2003, p. 6) more recent events of displacements, violations, and injustices can awaken with ferocity.

This is the danger of social traumas: We are pulled in by a force field and can lose our psychic footings. As we detangle that field, identifications can dislodge, and we can be stripped to a place we did not imagine, the "canvas" of our collective identifications threatening to fray (Volkan, 2001). There is always the risk that we will no longer be recognizable to ourselves. What was disavowed and dissociated can thaw and what we have known to be true can be infused with doubt. This, of course, is the place where psychic change might enter, if the therapeutic and/or communal scaffolding are present. But that was not the mandate at this truth commission.

Defining a witnessing presence

Our lives become predestined by the social forces that pull us in and by the social traumas that define how we are viewed and, more dangerously, how we view ourselves. This is a cloud that hovers, most urgently, over those living in zones where social violence becomes so "radioactive" (Gampel, 2000) that they are rendered almost impotent in the inhalation of its destructive elements. The psychologist working in this spiral has to take into account overlapping realities that are externally feeding an internal vortex. She has to try not to drown in the undertow, to hold onto humanity through a river of torment, culture, and confusion. This attempt to grasp for psychological truth is a form of witnessing that, according to Dori Laub (2007), seeks to document the "virtual internal truth," to record, in this case, the subjective experience of living with the unresolved and ongoing traumas of unacknowledged historical and current injustices. Chana Ullman's description of the psychologist–social witness' role engaging this field, is enormously helpful:

> Unlike the witness in a court of law who is expected to report the facts, the social witness is more effective in telling what it feels like, in uncovering what it means to be subjected to these conditions of suffering and evil (Margalit, 2002, Feldman and Laub, 1992, Ullman, 2006). Legal testimony provides evidence. It is followed by an attempt to judge among different versions of the truth; in moral witnessing, I believe the heart of the matter is that there is no version of the truth. The heart of the matter is that the social reality of suffering and evil is denied. This is, I believe, a fundamental condition for social witnessing: It begins where denial reigns.
>
> (2011, p. 186–7)

I want to echo what Ullman writes: "The heart of the matter is that the social reality of suffering and evil is denied." It is here that we face the mandate to give voice to what has been disavowed in the form of advocacy, and it is here that we have a potential role to play in accompanying those whose humanity has been denied (Roth and Duaibis, 2015). It is a project, as Frosh writes, that is inherently political carrying the

> injunction to face reality (that) reaches beyond the language of values and ideals and instead defines an attitude and approach that involves searching out whatever there is—however destructive, painful, guilt-inducing or shameful that may be, however much it impugns the good name of the individual or the society—however much that might then place on us a responsibility for difficult actions.
>
> (Frosh, 2007, p. 35)

It is from this space of social witnessing that we as clinicians might engage a specific kind of advocacy that includes: an amplification of the voices of those caught in the storm of social traumas, a highlighting of the psychological reverberations of the injustices that they must endure, and a consciousness-raising appeal that reaches to those in positions of influence.

Psychoanalytically informed clinicians can bring a particular clinical acumen to these battlegrounds, according to Pumla Gobodo-Madikizela, the South African psychologist who has written extensively on bearing witness and understanding evil (2003; 2013, personal communication).[6] Clinicians often have an ability to quickly connect the dots of what is dissociated and disavowed, a grasp of what systems are being activated or shut down, and an understanding of how impossible it is for people to engage and transform when flooded by guilt and/or shame. But we too struggle with an awareness that the lines between victim, perpetrator, bystander, and beneficiary are thin, sometimes even fluid; with an understanding that even those who have been involved in politically motivated atrocities are human; and with knowing that acknowledgment and accountability must be starting points for any healing process. Our vicarious traumatization may be our most important port of entry (Hirsch, 2003; Boulanger, 2013a) into the worlds of those on a frontline. Yet, we carry the liabilities of our countertransference, too—the internalized racism, marginality, shame, and the capacities for dissociation. And so we, too, can easily loose our footing.

Necessary disclosure

In a beautiful passage, Weingarten (2000, 2010) who has written extensively about bearing witness in conflict zones, captures the essence of how social trauma seeps into the present. Invoking the words of Antje Krog, a journalist who covered the Truth and Reconciliation hearings in South Africa, where witnessing meant seeing, "the arteries of our past bleed their own peculiar rhythm, tone and image" (Krog, 1998, p. 51), Weingarten reflects on how Krog loses her words in the face of so much sorrow and must face the ultimate dilemma: "If I write this, I exploit and betray. If I don't, I die" (Weingarten, 2000, p. 393; Krog, 1998, p. 66). Weingarten is highlighting the terrible quagmire all witnesses face: Are the stories we hear ours to tell? And can we turn what we have learned into knowledge, our own knowledge?[7]

Trying to describe realities that are multi-dimensional, infinitely complex, to which I do not really belong, but do not-not belong either, is terribly difficult. On the Israel–Palestine slope, who possesses what and who has legitimate claims to what is a relentless worry. I feel the privilege to move freely, to reach others, and to write, and with that comes the risk of betraying or imposing what is not mine to impose.

As an outsider I might misread. Israelis and Palestinians born and raised in the region, living closer to the epicenters of violence, have different defenses not only for managing anguish but for finessing what for those more distant, might seem incomprehensible. Some might interpret intensities in this field, using a yardstick that fails to contextualize this frontline in relation to other zones of ongoing political violence. One Israeli colleague asks: "When you say you are writing about Israel–Palestine as an 'extreme situation,' extreme relative to what?" (Mukamel, 2014, personal communication). Her question goes to the heart of the politics of suffering: Who defines what is extreme or a crisis? Who is more entitled to what because of their suffering, whose suffering is acknowledged or rendered invisible, whose is manipulated, whose goes underground? And, who gets to present it?

From the center of a vortex, radiating out

Scene I: a mother

Sami was one of the first people I met when I started learning about families living with political violence in East Jerusalem. He was my translator across cultures and language, the guide par excellence, the village historian, my bodyguard, in some respects, and the gatekeeper. He was also the reluctant host to the world of Palestinian women. It was only at the end of many days that he trusted me enough to introduce me to Amal, a meeting that opened a world and a search to understand.

Amal was an older mother, with one set of kids already out of the house and her youngest two, eight and ten years of age, at home. She talked about losing the will to parent. It was a simple and sad statement but incredibly powerful, because she was a woman whose energy and warmth broke through her walls of depression, nonetheless. As she talked, I found myself with reveries about 9/11, nursing my infant late at night, and the terrifying moments of nihilism. There was something about this first meeting, an evening in a home in a village, sitting around the living room, mattresses piled high to the side, grape leaves, and cookies with tea on the table and children on the floor drawing that was harrowing. The discrepancy between the warm, traditional hospitality that suggested normalcy and the threat of violence commingled in ways that were simultaneously organic but also suggestive of wildly discrepant realities that might be impossible to traverse.

Throughout the first part of our conversation, Sami translated, coaching me to eat, lest I insult Amal. But at some point it became clear that he was not conveying the essence of what I was saying, and a gap developed between what I thought I was asking, what he was asking, and what Amal was saying. Finally, I asked him if he was translating, and he said no. He said he was worried that I would lead this mother into talking too much about her pain. Could I talk about something "pink," a word that had become code between us, for color and hope. The day before, when Sami had described how everything in his village had become black and white, how people had lost their appetite for certain pleasures, he said that he "longed to see pink." Was he afraid of hearing Amal's anguish and claims? Perhaps he was protecting her from me, my modernity, or maybe he needed to control Amal from expressing too much or from reaching a larger public, as the twinned social tensions of patriarchy and occupation are always on the backs of women here (Tonsern, 2011). But I now wonder if Sami was shielding himself or Amal not just from pain and longing, but from what might come after her pain.

Amal and I locked eyes, as if we both knew that something was awry. I walked over to her and using my hands, asked her if we could keep talking; if it was okay. She nodded, or so I remember, and I continued: I said that I just wanted to hear what she had to say and only what she wanted to tell me, and if it feels too dark, she should let me know. Somehow, and I still do not know how, she and I did the rest of the interview in gestures. She was concerned about her children and grandchildren but worried about how distracted she could become. She was a different mother for her younger children then she had been for her older children, now parents themselves. She was preoccupied, too tired to contain her children's aggression or to enforce the discipline needed to help them get to school, stay out of trouble. She worried that she would not be able to keep them in line and channel their energies effectively. I learned that she was living with a kind of anticipatory terror, that her home would be taken away or demolished and that her children might be inducted into a world of violence, an adolescent rite of passage for some teens in the community. She touched her heart and somehow conveyed, "You are a mother too," implying that I would understand.

Amal's message was clear and visceral: I am worried about maintaining my home, I am worried my children, and I am trying to make a life in the midst, and my mind is preoccupied, scrambled at times. I am not able to contain my anger as well as I used too. And I am tired.

Amal brings us into the center of a storm, the ways in which social traumas penetrate the very private, intimate worries of a mother and hijack the ability to calmly bear in mind what a mother needs to bear in mind. She raises the issue of how we are both "affected" and "infected" by social trauma (Heyno, 2008; Cohen, 2015),[8] how terrifying it is to lose our abilities to parent, to feel deep maternal meaning, and to serve as protective shields for our children. Her story raises questions about how this particular political violence reverberates into family living, and it resonates with what Shalhoub-Kevorkian writes: Palestinian mothers and children are "frontliners," incurring the "first wave of violence, as well as the final one" (2009, p. 4). Meeting Amal ignited a course of engagement that revolved around the following question: What kind of witnessing presence, if any, can we bring to families living in zones of protracted conflict? Might there be a form of presence that can lessen irrevocable damage? And, can we reach for subjective truths that might infuse human rights advocacy?

Scene II

A soft-spoken Palestinian man, a father of four children, walks with a small group through his village. His home smells like "skunk water," a foul smelling liquid that was sprayed through the windows during one of the weekly demonstrations. The stench is wretched. He talks about the "mapping" of the neighborhoods, a word that is meant to describe a process in which children are photographed so as to later aid in their identification and arrest. The word "mapping" lingers. It is a word I used often in my office when I would talk to patients about mapping their visions or longings. But now the word is twisted, as the brutality it references is normalized by this euphemism. Much later, I will write that "neighborhoods are mapped," no longer feeling my first shock and revulsion. I will render these words as non-emotional facts, the violence in some way normalized, which is precisely the issue in these trenches. A journalist I met during that first walking orientation to these villages had asked, "At what moments does a child become a child in the eyes of soldier?" And I thought, "Maybe never," and then wrote in my notes, "What will it take to keep a child, 'a child' in our minds? And, what will it take to keep a mother, a mother?"

The dangers of desensitization and dehumanization lurk when words like "mapping" are used euphemistically and normalized. But what dangers lurk when terrible knowledge is not normalized? That is, are there dangers in trying to hold conflicting realities and managing immense cognitive dissonance?

Reflection: psychoanalytic presence

A colleague asks: Once you have been in the field to bear witness is it really necessary to go again? Don't you know enough already? And doesn't your presence retraumatize those who might be compelled to tell stories, unaware of how the retelling might trigger traumas that are beyond symbolization? Similarly, another colleague wonders about the implicit pessimism in bearing witness in a zone of ongoing political conflict: Isn't bearing witness a stance that reflects a "last hope" of what we might offer in the face of ongoing brutality, signaling defeat in changing an existing order? Shouldn't our aspirations as mental health practitioners aim higher, toward changing systems of injustice while intervening with more aggressive projects that humanize and provide healing (Greenbaum, 2015, personal communication)?

Do psychologists have any place in trying to imagine a more human and humane response? These questions go to the heart of this chapter: Is witnessing in a zone of ongoing conflict a good idea? Is it helpful and, to whom?

Concerns are legitimate: Witnessing is always complex. But there remains the possibility that our presence, if desired, might provide a form of "psychological accompaniment" (Watkins, 2012), enabling survivors to bring to life that which has been fractured and dissociated, as they wrestle with us, the proxies for all those who have turned away. Reno Papadopoulos calls this a form of "therapeutic witnessing," through which stakeholders might "re-story" and "restore" themselves—as they "re-member" (2002, p. 34). It is a dynamic presence that may sow the seeds for, what Weingarten calls, "reasonable hope," a hope that can derive from having unrecognized trauma validated and from having one's efforts at living with dignity, acknowledged (Weingarten, 2010). Amplification of the micro ways in which survivors lay claim to their humanity, without negating the vast injustices they face, is a crucial means of generating energy and meaning.

Our cannon of psychoanalytic and psychological literature reminds us that holding environments, attachment relationships, and social supports foster a capacity to tolerate and adapt to painful life experiences, buffering against the potentially adverse effects of ongoing trauma (Freud and Burlingham, 1943; Winnicott, 1965; Bowlby, 1969) and activating the capacity to reflect on experience and witness the self (Fonagy and Target, 1997; Weingarten, 2003). Might we then think about our role as witnesses to social trauma as a small step toward defusing the toxicity of extreme environments, not just once the war is over but during it as well?

At the same time, can we hold a "deep respect for extreme environments," as Lifton says (see Chapter 9, this volume), perhaps a cautionary warning that engaging those who live in hazardous and unpredictable terrains should be approached soberly? Research from this region suggests that even the best of holding environments—the best parent–child dyads—cannot maintain their protective function in the face of external forces of violence (Quota, Punamaki, and El Sarraj, 2005). By extension, the same might be true for the limits of the holding and containment that a ring of witnesses might provide.

Scene III: a child

I want to listen to the boy I can barely remember, who shared the story of his arrest and detention and how his deep worry about his mother haunted him throughout. His twelve-year-old sister, dressed in her school uniform, sat near him, captivated by his account. When I grasp just why I cannot remember this boy, he comes back in full color: His name is Jamal, and his story was the not the worst story I had heard. I interviewed him in his living room with a close colleague of mine and with a Holocaust scholar. As with Amal, the civility of a living room that could have been anywhere was harrowing: It was the most normal of "normals," except we were in a refugee camp and were told that almost every night there were night raids and the arrest of teenage boys. As a mother then of a teenage boy, roughly the same age, whose younger sister hung on his every word, I could not bear the similarity in the family composition and dynamics.

Jamal relayed a story about being awakened in the middle of the night by soldiers, of thinking that he would escape this experience, and of his dismay that he hadn't. He honed in on how his mother was "screaming, going hysterical, crying." The words of another teenager came to mind: He too worried about his mother, while he was in detention and longed to be with her. I wonder if these adolescents worry about their mothers' pain, because their mothers link them to the birth of being human? Perhaps, the most primal call for "mother" comes in the confrontation with death and the breakdown of civility (Davoine and Gaudilliere, 2004)? And, perhaps the primal longing for one's children comes as we see them skidding toward that edge? Through their mothers' eyes, they might see the erosion of their own humanity and the moral injuries they have endured. Their experience of dehumanization, as victim or perpetrator or both, may then become more transparent and accessible (Shay, 1994). In an agonizing testimony from Breaking the Silence,[9] an Israeli soldier painfully describes how he finally understood what he did to Palestinian families when he raided their homes during his army service. He tells an interviewer that his guilt and shame became intolerable while he and his mother watched video footage he shot while on duty, and he saw what he did through his mother's eyes. If mothering might be partially construed as reminding children who they are existentially, might it also be construed as reminding them of who they are not?

Jamal recalled one other detail as he told his story: The soldiers seemed sorry for what was happening, and his mother told us: "The soldiers were actually trying to be gentle." No one can stand the anguish between mothers and children, is what I scribbled. In retrospect, Jamal and his mother's abilities to see and hold onto the soldiers' humanity seem remarkable. How were they able to remember this tenderness in the face of what must have felt assaultive? Is it possible that the eyes of a mother, in addition to tracking the erosion of humanity, might also carry the need to seek out the humane, even in the face of brutality?

Reflection: psychoanalytic presence as problematic

At times, I hear Palestinian colleagues posing the following concerns about psychoanalytic modes of listening and engaging and their relevance to those living with political violence: Might these modes of engagement encourage stakeholders to become "too soft," too open to longings and disappointments to then manage the trials of daily reality? Could our psychoanalytically informed witnessing evoke too much pain and hope by arousing visions for realities that will never find expression? Additionally, might this softness interfere with the much needed energy and determination to resist oppressive policies?

These concerns go to the very heart of a difficult issue for psychoanalysts: Do we underestimate the psychological dangers that lurk if we encourage people living in zones of injustice to engage their inner worlds? While witnessing may facilitate the "repossession" of a life story bringing profound validation (Boulanger, 2014), there are risks for those we accompany in awakening dreams for that which cannot exist and in feeling what might be too devastating too feel.

"Nur," a young Palestinian mother living in a neighborhood facing continuous night-time incursions, was terrified that her nine-year-old son might be arrested for allegedly throwing stones. She stopped our first meeting to tend to her elderly father and our second was in the company of children seeking help with homework. When I asked her what gave her strength, she talked about the joys of her youth, the greater access she had to pleasurable activities and outings. And then she relayed the following: Not long ago, her elderly father had spotted a hole in her pants. She believed that "it killed him" to see her degraded, and so he went out to buy her new ones without saying a word. Deeply appreciative of her father's wish to protect her and restore her dignity, she associated to wanting another honeymoon and reflected proudly on how she built her home with her own hands, a kitchen that had two buckets for a sink. But soon her powerful fears intruded, and she began ruminating that all her labor would be destroyed and her home demolished. My question triggered a rapid loop that included a memory of restored dignity, then desire and pride, then terror. As we closed this interchange, Nur asked me to check the safety of medication she was prescribed for anxiety. Her agitation had returned, and with it, our joint deflation.

Can we, as engaged outsiders, work with the inevitable seduction and disappointments we trigger? Could our witnessing lead to an easing of coping strategies and an unleashing of powerful frustrations? Might those of us raised and trained in a milieu more removed from the threats of our own personal annihilation be less attuned to how our more active engagements could be problematic in the face of pressing social trauma? Ullman raises a related, pressing concern: As we witness, do we help people awaken to their rage so as to fight oppressive systems, or do we help them quiet their rage, encouraging them to make peace with injustice (Ullman, 2009)? What guarantees can we provide that reaching forward, deeply, and intimately toward their psychic centers might support creative resistance to injustice? And, as Samah Jabr writes, are we really able to hear the ramifications of prolonged repressive and oppressive policies, when we ourselves are the beneficiaries of the system that oppresses (Jabr and Berger, 2015)?

Psychoanalytic formulating empowers us with powerful thinking tools but simultaneously runs the risk of "othering." It is not easy to resist the seduction of a psychoanalytic lens that imbues meaning and, hence, claims victory by interpreting. When I can think about how the collapsing of dimensionality and individual uniqueness is enacted repeatedly on this frontline, how everyone is trying to occupy everyone else, to lay claim, cross boundaries, control, and erase, I feel stronger. When I describe how the rejected other is not only invisible but is rendered undesirable, hated, where the only solution is violent dispossession, I feel a sense of triumph of having named *the* toxin. But I know this triumph is suspect. It is too hard to admit my wordlessness in the face of the other who is flattened by oppression, because it reveals my own nihilism that threatens to defeat (Roth, 2011).

Outer rims of the witnessing circles

Palestinian, Israeli, and international human rights workers both locally and internationally bear the burdens of living with political turmoil themselves. Those on the Palestinian–Israeli frontline inhale the impact of a system that normalizes harsh measures to prevent resistance. One Palestinian worker, relaying her own experiences as a child said, "It was routine for soldiers to come in the middle of the night. But now it has hit me that I grew up with night raids," a term and concept she had never used, and never really conceptualized as abnormal. "If I were to think how terrible it was, I wouldn't have survived. You need to stop seeing things the way they are." Disavowal is a needed survival strategy that might drain the event of its intensity but also keeps daily life moving.

At some point, humanitarian workers cross a threshold and are likely to get hurt by the social traumas in which they too live. As responders, they are witnesses whose stories and anguish are not acknowledged sufficiently and are thus at risk for vicarious traumatization. One international humanitarian worker remarked that she was fine until the bubble around her began to tear: "I don't know when it was, maybe two or three years after I started living here. I started seeing what was underneath the surface. It wasn't a conscious decision. But once I saw it, I could not, not see it anymore. And then things got very difficult."

For aid workers from abroad, there is perhaps a fantasy, coupled by the expectations from locals, that their passports and privileges should exempt them from pain and protect them from harassment. And, by comparison, maybe they do to some extent. But these privileges do not protect enough.[10] Many are left alone to navigate the crossing of literal and figurative borders. One international human rights worker articulated the following:

> We witness the human rights violations and the oppression. The fear I have is looking at it as a normal situation … I've gotten more distressed living with situations I cannot changed: I can't fly over a checkpoint … I have the right passport. I can cross. But there is a feeling that I will have to argue with them (soldiers). It's stressful. It has an impact knowing that I'm privileged just because the system of oppression is set up that way. It's a system that segregates people. I belong to the side that's privileged … The main problem is your daily life with the constant problem of having to deal with soldiers, police, checkpoints, problems with visas. We can't really tell people at the border crossings what we are doing here, even though we have been sent by our governments. So there is an impact of your situation not being secured, of having to finesse the situation. If anything does happen, there really isn't anyone to protect you. We are documenting the worsening of a situation. We are bystanders to a de-developing situation that is intolerable.

These workers share the terrible knowledge—almost impossible to say out loud, lest their pain eclipse the pain of Palestinians who are the direct targets of oppressive policies—that they too are pulled into a spiraling field of injustices that have been normalized, where anguish is rendered invisible.

> We can't really speak. We are ashamed by the suffering we feel, but can it be acknowledged? Another added: There's a point where there's

> irreversible damage: While we all get more cynical, that cynicism is a coping mechanism and won't stay permanently. But there does seem to be a threshold that once it's pushed, will make it difficult to go back.

Outsiders, who are not raised in this particular political turmoil, may not be inoculated to the specific traumatic contagions and so are at risk. But these outsiders give a powerful emotional reading of the damaging impact of the political and social violence specific to this region.

Discussion

As this chapter comes to a close, I feel the vast distance between the lives of those living in this field of continuous traumatic stress and those of us further away. No matter how much we subscribe to "being more human than otherwise," and no matter how much we might tell ourselves that it is fate that put us on one side of the divide versus another, or that it is fate that has us carrying one legacy versus another, we still have to reckon with our privilege, our near escape from a similar destiny, our freedoms and "their" imprisonments. It raises the complex question of what it means for us to "discuss," while others "suffer"—for us to use words, grasp for metaphors, and to even pause, while lives are propelled with unpredictable force into an unknown and possibly dangerous future. It begs the question, why not activism, policy, or human rights advocacy instead? Why our thoughts as therapists? What will it feel like for those in the region to be written about? Have I run the risk of appropriating and imposing meaning?

But maybe there is no way to avoid these dangers and, in fact, to enact them, unless we too are silenced? The issue of being dispossessed or erased is the current that runs from the lives of those at the epicenter of these concentric fields—the children, Palestinian and Israeli, who are inducted into a world of militarism that endangers their homes, communities, and futures—all the way to those at the edges. Whose history and whose lives matter, and whose must go underground? And what dangers lurk when violence is normalized, when people know—but do not know—terrible things, and then live in conflicting realities managing immense cognitive dissonance?

Along these circles there is compassion fatigue, a worry about losing meaning—maternal meaning, professional meaning, and the deepest meaning of all—what you know to be true of yourself. The fear that social traumas define the self and twist it echoes. I believe this might be at the heart of the dangers of dispossession and internalized tribalism. These are the ripples of trauma that cut across the radius of these concentric circles.

Perhaps, the eyes of the maternal witness, real or imagined, protect? Perhaps, placing children at the heart of the epicenter of this storm instructs, reminding us that social traumas bear down on the next generations? Maybe the primal call for the mother and the primal call for one's children come, as we skid toward the breakdowns of civilization? Maybe an ethic of care, as Carol Gilligan writes, "in its concern for voice and relationships" and in its focus on the dangers of thoughtlessness, disrespect, and silencing (Gilligan, 2014, p. 90)—that are at the very heart of relational psychoanalysis—invite a new ethic of human rights? From this perspective, human rights violations are psychological ruptures, where the wounds of war and moral trauma are defined, as Jessica Benjamin (2014) writes, as betrayals of what we are relationally primed to trust—that we can be justly heard and believed, so that some realities do not have the power to erase other realities.

If psychoanalytic presence might be construed as the referring of demons and competing identifications (Rozmarin, 2010; Frosh, 2013), psychological accompaniment might be the process of defining those forces that presently demonize by bringing them into a shared, safe space where fears, shame, and alienation and pain can be held. Psychoanalysts enrich the process of psychological accompaniment because we grasp that to really "see" anguish, means to feel and know a place that often defies symbolization, challenging core beliefs and identity. We might help open spaces that can contain reflection (Long, personal communication, 2014), and partner in creating webs of concerned professionals who can amplify and responsibly disseminate terrible realities in ways that ignite reasonable hope, that in the midst of all that might suggest otherwise, there is still life in these trenches.[11] Our presence in a zone of ongoing political violence might be construed as a form of standing in solidarity, of leveling the playing field, of partnering and engaging—all in the effort of "communalizing" the traumas (Shay, 1994) and reaching for a "moral third," where there is an acknowledgment of violations and ruptures in what is right (Benjamin, 2014). This form of responsive witnessing could entail seeing and holding individual and collective pain and genuine liveliness and, with that, supporting the quest for rectifying justice through collaborative projects. This is what Ad-Dab'agh calls "compassionate witnessing," rooted in the maternal capacities of loyalty, containment, and "being with" (Ad-Dab'agh, 2015).

If the silence in the face of dispossession is finally given voice, the ability to acknowledge the perpetrator and even our own complicity as bystanders given space, might there be some prayer in preventing the transmission of the unarticulated shadows to the next generation? Psychological accompaniment might be some small measure toward prevention.

Finally, listening to the individual and collective voices from zones of continuous trauma is humbling and instructive. It changes what we experience in our offices and what we see in our own communities by highlighting how racism and tribalism penetrate the psyche, by pointing to the kinds of relational and communal safeguards necessary to withstand these social ills, and by teaching us what it takes to "survive hating and being hated" (White, 2002), to resist it creatively, and to maintain dignity in its face.

Notes

1 Lederech (2005) lightly refers to witnesses, attuned to the ways in which injustice tears at the fabric of their community, as "dwellers at the threshold," a metaphor he borrows from a Van Morrison song (1982).
2 See Watkins (2012) and Rodriguez et al. (2009).
3 Slade nests mentalization in concentric circles (Slade, personal communication, 2010); in gratitude to A. Slade and J. Mathews for helping to visualize the transmission of psychic pain across concentric fields (personal communication, 2012). See also Tripplehorn and Chen (2006).
4 See Frosh (2013) on how trauma is "vertically" transmitted across generations and "horizontally" transmitted across the complexity of the relational field. See Boulanger (2013b) for contagion effects of social and environmental traumas.
5 Zochrot, Truth Commission, December 10, 2014, addressing the years 1948–1960 in Southern Israel (http://zochrot.org/en/content/17, accessed July 6, 2016).
6 The following authors' work on witnessing has collectively been powerfully instructive: Boulanger (2007; 2008; 2013; 2014), Weingarten (2000; 2010), and Gerson (2009).
7 Grateful to M. Zak for this insight.
8 Cohen applies Heyno's concept of being affected and infected to the realm of social trauma.
9 See http://born-equal.net/blog/2012/05/16/arrest-of-a-15-years-old-an-israeli-soldiers-testimony-breaking-the-silence-april-2011/, accessed July 6, 2016.
10 Foreign aid workers all over the world are put in danger psychologically (see Global Psychosocial Network http://www.globalpsychosocialnetwork.org; Weyderman, 2010), and that is no less true in Israel–Palestine.
11 In gratitude to Born Equal (http://born-equal.net), the Global Psychosocial Network, Psychologists for Social Responsibility, and the once Mental Health Activists in Partnership, who creatively engage advocacy, accompaniment, and witnessing.

References

Ad-Dab'bagh, Y. (2015). Compassionate witnessing in the face of erasure: A commentary on crows on the cradles: Palestinian mothers at a frontline vortex: Reflections on the psychology of occupation by Judy Roth and Salwa Duaibis. *International Journal of Applied Psychoanalytical Studies*, 12(3):295–303.

Benjamin, J. (2014). The discarded and the dignified. http://www.publicseminar.org/2014/12/the-discarded-and-the-dignified-parts-1-and-2/#.VQJHuMa3w21, accessed July 6, 2016.

Boulanger, G. (2007). *Wounded by reality: Understanding and treating adult onset trauma*. Hillsdale: Analytic Press.

Boulanger, G. (2008). Witnesses to reality: Working psychodynamically with survivors of terror. *Psychoanalytic Dialogues*, 18(5):638–657.

Boulanger, G. (2013a). Fearful symmetry: Shared trauma in New Orleans after Hurricane Katrina. *Psychoanalytic Dialogues*, 23(1):31–44.

Boulanger, G. (2013b). Vicarious trauma: A necessary therapeutic tool. Paper delivered at City University of New York.

Boulanger, G. (2014). The continuing and unfinished present: Oral history and psychoanalysis in the aftermath of terror. In Cave, M. and Sloan, S. (Eds.), *Listening on the edge: Oral history in the aftermath of crisis*. Oxford: Oxford University Press.

Bowlby, J. (1969). *Attachment*. Attachment and loss (vol. 1). New York: Basic Books.

Cohen, E. (2015). Opening remarks: Intergenerational attachment patterns and the responses of child therapists in the presence of societal trauma. International Association Relational Psychoanalysis and Psychotherapy, Webinar, March 14, 2015.

Davoine, F. and Gaudilliere, J. (2004). *History beyond trauma: Whereof one cannot speak, thereof one cannot stay silent*. New York: Other Press.

Even-Tzur, E. (2016). "The road to the village": The Israeli social unconscious and the Palestinian Nakba, *International Journal of Applied Psychoanalytic Studies*. http://onlinelibrary.wiley.com/doi/10.1002/aps.1478/, accessed July 6, 2016.

Feldman, S. and Laub, D. (1992). *Testimony: Crises of witnessing in literature, psychoanalysis, and history*. New York: Routledge.

Fonagy, P. and Target, M. (1996). Playing with reality: I. Theory of mind and the normal development of psychic reality. *International Journal of Psycho-Analysis*, 77(2):217–233.

Freud, A. and Burlingham, D. (1943). *War and children*. New York: Medical War Books.

Frosh, S. (2007). Facing political truths. *Psychotherapy and Politics International*, 5(1):29–37.

Frosh, S. (2013). *Hauntings: Psychoanalysis and ghostly transmissions.* Basingstoke: Palgrave Macmillan.

Gampel, Y. (2000). The prevalence of the uncanny in social violence. In Robben, A. and Suarez-Orozco, M. (Eds). *Cultures under siege: Collective violence and trauma.* Cambridge: Cambridge University Press.

Gerson, S. (2009). When the third is dead: Memory, mourning, and witnessing in the aftermath of the Holocaust. *International Journal of Psychoanalysis*, 90(6):1341–1357.

Gilligan, C. (2014). Moral injury and the ethic of care: Reframing the conversation about differences. *Journal of Social Philosophy*, 45(1):89–106.

Gobodo-Madikizela, P. (2003). *A human being died that night: A South African woman confronts the legacy of apartheid.* New York: Houghton Mifflin.

Goren, E.R. and Alpert, J.L. (this volume). The analyst as witness, historian and activist: A conversation with Robert Jay Lifton. In Alpert, J.L. and Goren, E.R. (Eds). *Psychoanalysis, trauma, and community: History and contemporary reappraisals.* Relational Perspectives book series, L. Aron and A. Harris, series editors.

Grob, L. (2016). Torture during the holocaust: Responsible witnessing. In Grob, L. and Roth, J. K. (Eds). *Losing trust in the world: Holocaust scholars confront torture.* Stephen S. Weinstein Series in Post-Holocaust Studies. Seattle: University of Washington Press.

Hamber, B. (2009). *Transforming societies after political violence: Truth, reconciliation, and mental health.* New York: Springer.

Heyno, A. (2008). One being affected without being infected: Managing suicidal thoughts in student counseling. In Briggs, S., Lemma, A. and Crouch, W. (Eds). *Related to self-harm and suicide: Psychoanalytic perspectives on practice, theory, and prevention.* London: Routledge.

Hirsch, I. (2003). Reflections on clinical issues in the context of the national trauma of September 11. *Contemporary Psychoanalysis*, 39(4):665–681.

Hoffman, E. (2004). *After such knowledge: Memory, history, and the legacy of the Holocaust.* New York: Public Affairs.

Jabr, S. and Berger, E. (2015). An occupied state of mind: Clinical transference and countertransference across the Israeli/Palestinian divide. *Psychoanalysis, Culture & Society*, 21(4):21–40.

Keilson, H. (1992). *Sequential traumatization in children: A clinical and statistical follow-up study of the fate of Jewish war orphans in the Netherlands.* Jerusalem: Magnes Press.

Krog, A. (1998). *Country of my skull: Guilt, sorry, and the limits of forgiveness in the new South Africa.* Johannesburg: Random House South Africa.

Krog, A. (2000). *Country of my skull: Guilt, sorrow, and the limits of forgiveness in the new South Africa.* New York: Three Rivers Press.

Laub, D. (2007). Not knowing is an active process of destruction. Why the testimonial procedure is of so much importance. *Special Review Issue*, Newsletter, 2.

Lederch, J.P. (2005). *The moral imagination: The art and soul of building peace*. New York: Oxford University Press.

Margalit, A. (2002). *The ethics of memory*. Cambridge: Harvard University Press.

Oliver, M. (2015). *Felicity*. New York: Penguin Press.

Papadopoulos, R.K. (2002). Refugees home and trauma. In Papadopoulos, R.K. (Ed.), *Therapeutic care for refugees: No place like home*. London: Karnac.

Quota, S., Punamaki, R.L. and El Sarraj, E. (2005). Mother-child expression of psychological distress in war trauma. *Clinical Child Psychology and Psychiatry*, 10:135–156.

Rodriguez, S.S., Guerra, C.T., Villareal, L.F.G. and Bohorques, R.V. (2009). Psychological accompaniment: Construction of cultures of peace among a community affected by war. In M. Montero and C.C. Sonn (Eds). *Psychology of Liberation*. Peace Psychology Book Series, 221. New York: Springer Science & Business Media.

Roth, J. (2011). The arc of a frontline. *The Psychoanalytic Activist*, October.

Roth, J. and Duaibis, S. (2015). Crows on the cradles: Palestinian mothers at a frontline vortex—reflections on the psychology of occupation. *International Journal of Applied Psychoanalytic Studies*, 12(1):5–20.

Rozmarin, E. (2010). Better identity politics. *Psychoanalytic Dialogues*, 20(2):181–190.

Shalhoub-Kevorkian, N. (2009). *Militarization and violence against women in conflict zones in the Middle East: A Palestinian case-study (Cambridge studies in law and society)*. New York: Cambridge University Press.

Shay, J. (1994). *Achilles in Vietnam: Combat trauma and the undoing of character*. New York: Scribner.

Tonsern, M. (2011). *Palästinensische frauen zwischen besatzung und patriarchat – eine kulturwissenschaftliche Analyse [Palestinian women between occupation and patriarchy—an analysis]*. Graz: Leykam Verlag.

Tripplehorn, C. and Chen, C. (2006). Layers of support: The social ecology of protecting children in war. In Boothby, N., Strang, A. and Wessells, M.A. (Eds). *A world turned upside down: Social-ecological approaches to children in war zones*. West Hartford: Kumarian Press.

Ullman, C. (2006). Bearing witness: Across the barriers in society and in the clinic. *Psychoanalytic Dialogues*, 16(2):181–198.

Ullman, C. (2009). Opening post, "The trauma of morality," International Association Relational Psychoanalysis and Psychotherapy Colloquium Series, No. 14, May 11, 2009.

Ullman, C. (2011) Between denial and witnessing: Psychoanalysis and clinical practice in the Israeli context. *Psychoanalytic Perspectives*, 8(2):179–200.

Volkan, V. (2001). Transgenerational transmissions and chosen traumas: An aspect of large-group identity. *Group Analysis*, 34(1):79–97.

Watkins, M. (2012). Accompaniment: Psychosocial, environmental, trans-species, earth. Plenary panel for Psychologists for Social Responsibility in Washington, DC, July 13.

Weingarten, K. (2000). Witnessing, wonder, and hope. *Family Process*, 39(4):389–402.

Weingarten, K. (2003). Compassionate witnessing and the transformation of societal violence: How individuals can make a difference. Manuscript adapted with permission from *Common Shock*, London: Penguin.

Weingarten, K. (2010). Reasonable hope: Construct, clinical applications, and supports. *Family Process*, 49(1):5–25.

Weyderman, B. (2010). *Close encounters: Stories from the frontline of human rights work in Nepal*. Nepal: Himal Books.

White, K.P. (2002). Surviving hating and being hated: Some personal thoughts about racism from a psychoanalytic perspective. *Contemporary Psychoanalysis*, 38(3):401–422.

Winnicott, D.W. (1965). *Maturational processes and the facilitating environment: Studies in the theory of emotional development*. London: Hogwarth Press.

Zochrot website: http://zochrot.org/en/content/17.

Part II

Therapeutic encounters outside the frame

Chapter 3

The multiple traumas of Hurricane Katrina as witnessed by a psychoanalytic first responder[1]

Laurel Bass Wagner

Introduction

Hurricane Katrina made landfall in southeastern Louisiana at 6:10 a.m. August 29, 2005. Less than 24 hours earlier, New Orleans mayor Ray Nagin ordered the first-ever mandatory evacuation of the city. For those with few or no resources it was too late. Residents in care facilities throughout the region relied on buses that never came. Thirty-one residents of St. Rita's Nursing in St. Bernard Parish died, primarily from drowning. The city established "refuges of last resort," such as the Superdome, to shelter citizens who could not leave. The Superdome was badly damaged by the hurricane, leaving its occupants stranded with little or no food, water, and electricity and few bathroom facilities. The storm surge caused 53 levee breaches, resulting in the worst civil engineering disaster in US history. Eighty percent of New Orleans, and large portions of neighboring parishes, were submerged. It was the third deadliest natural disaster and the largest diaspora in US history, with 1,836 lives lost, 35,000 rescued and 1.7 million displaced (Picou and Marshall, 2007). Three hundred thousand homes were lost, ten times more than any other natural disaster in the country. The economic damage was more than 100 billion dollars, making it the costliest natural disaster in US history. No statistic, however, can quantify the magnitude of human suffering caused by the hurricane, flooding, and the subsequent inadequate responses of the local, state, and federal governments.

I have provided mental health disaster relief for over 20 years, responding to airplane crashes, mass shootings, and natural disasters. Five hundred miles from the disaster site I encountered the largest disaster of my career: 50,000 New Orleanians evacuated to Dallas, Texas. As a mental health first responder I assisted the evacuees who arrived in the direst of circumstances. These were the individuals who ended up in the Dallas Red Cross shelters between August 31 and September 15, 2005.

Thousands of New Orleans residents lacked the means, both literally and figuratively, to evacuate before the hurricane hit and the levees broke. The majority were African-American. Many were poor, under-educated, unemployed or underemployed, and disabled. In many respects the country had failed them long before it failed them in response to the hurricane. Their story is one of multiple traumas, which began long before Hurricane Katrina swept away the vestiges of anything that resembled normal life. For these individuals racial, ethnic, and/or class disparities formed the backdrop to the devastation of the hurricane and its aftermath. The question was often asked, either publicly or privately, "Why didn't they leave?" The answer, "They couldn't leave" can only be understood in the context of what Leary (2006) calls, "the realities attending generational poverty among the urban underclass" (p. 346). Those whose lives were the hardest prior to the hurricane were those who suffered the most in its aftermath. These were the people I met in the Dallas Red Cross shelters.

Theories of trauma

Victims of trauma find their worlds fundamentally altered. Hurricane Katrina destroyed the world of many New Orleanians. Their dwellings, streets, stores, schools, hospitals, and churches no longer existed; the city's infrastructure was gone. They lacked water, food, and shelter. For tens of thousands no help was forthcoming. The personal toll was even worse. Trust, if there in the first place, was breached. Likewise, attachments of all kinds—to family, friends, and community—were mangled. When all is lost the sense of self often experiences a collapse. Those left in New Orleans when the levees broke were lost in every sense of the word.

Prior to the disaster many of these individuals had already faced trauma in their lives. Some were homeless, mentally ill, or both. Some were the victims of abuse, violence, and drugs. Some were perpetrators of abuse and violence and some were both victims and perpetrators. The mentally ill and those with prior trauma histories are the most susceptible to developing acute stress disorders and posttraumatic stress disorders. In essence, those already compromised are the most traumatized (Muesser et al.,

1998; Kessler, 2000; North et al., 2004; Scott, 2007). Additionally, recent evidence suggests traumatic load (higher trauma exposure) may be the root cause of posttraumatic stress disorder (PTSD) chronicity and symptom severity (Kolassa et al., 2010).

How humans adapt and respond to traumatic stress is explained by a number of theories (see Benight, 2012 for a review). Three theories are particularly relevant to the Katrina evacuees in the Dallas Red Cross shelters. Attachment theory, a psychoanalytic theory of human development, postulates human beings develop attachments early in life because their lives depend on it (Bowlby, 1969). Identifiable, stable attachment patterns develop and are internalized as internal working models that determine access to thoughts, feeling, and memories related to attachment. Disruptions in these relationships create vulnerability in one's sense of self and others, and inhibit the capacity to contain and regulate affective experience (Slade, 2000). Individuals who go through life with insecure or disorganized attachments lack resilience and are susceptible to disruptions in the sense of self, especially in the face of trauma. The homeless, mentally ill, substance abusers, and/or victims of interpersonal trauma are much more likely to lack secure and/or stable attachments. In the face of disaster, those without secure attachments experience a decline in interpersonal and intrapsychic functioning that often results in stress symptoms and disorders (Carlson and Dallenberg, 2000; Benight, 2012). Many Katrina evacuees in the Dallas Red Cross shelters lacked the internal resources to help them cope and respond in a resilient way to the insults they suffered in response to the hurricane and its aftermath. The disaster left them with compromised senses of self, often overwhelmed by emotion. Moreover, the combined traumas of the hurricane, the failure of the levees, and the failure of the government to anticipate and adequately respond to the most basic needs of those stuck in New Orleans likely created not just a threatened sense of self, but a nearly demolished one.

The central tenet of Conservation of Resources (COR) Theory (Hobfoll, 1989, 1991) is that people strive to obtain, build, and protect what they value (their resources) and psychological stress occurs when their resources are lost or their loss is threatened. These resources may be possessions (for example home), personal characteristics (for example optimism), conditions (for example good relationships, financial security) and energies (for example time, knowledge). Hobfoll defines traumatic stress as the sudden, unpredictable loss of extensive resources. The individuals I encountered in the Dallas shelters experienced an almost total loss of resources as swiftly as the hurricane came and went. Even the clothes on their backs didn't belong to them. Natural disasters often involve a loss of resources, and the validity of this theory has been empirically documented, including among Hurricane Katrina survivors. Resource loss is positively associated with psychological distress, trauma symptoms, PTSD, and mental illness, with death of a relative and house destroyed among the most salient variables (Freedy et al., 1994; Calera et al., 2001; Sastry and VanLandingham, 2009).

Strozier (2002), in his work with victims of the attacks on the World Trade Center, conceptualizes individual reactions to trauma on a vertical and horizontal axis. I apply Strozier's theory to the Hurricane Katrina victims. The vertical axis represents the individual's prior experience of traumas to the self. The horizontal axis represents how close the individual was to "ground zero." The term "ground zero" was first used to describe the blast site of a nuclear weapon, with the blast radiating out in concentric circles of lessening destruction. This term immediately took hold to describe the center of violence at the World Trade Center. For Hurricane Katrina, ground zero is New Orleans where the levees broke and the neighborhoods were submerged. Strozier poetically describes "zones of sadness," which radiated in concentric circles from the Twin Towers site (p. 366). The closer to the site, the greater the sadness, which is exacerbated by prior trauma experiences in the individual. Strozier's theory is psychoanalytically grounded in its understanding of the cumulative effects of trauma.

Psychological first aid

The acute phase of work with trauma victims is called psychological first aid. From a psychoanalytic perspective this means shoring up defenses to promote resiliency, not exploration. That comes later when the self begins to reconstitute and regains the ability to reflect. Psychological first aid focuses on promoting a sense of safety, calmness, self and community efficacy, connectedness, and hope (Hobfoll et al., 2007; Vernberg et al., 2008). Boulanger (2005) describes how "the adult self collapses during massive trauma as the experience of agency, of affectivity, of physical cohesiveness and continuity are challenged by disassociation" (p. 22). Many Katrina victims were initially unable to tell their stories. They were numb, wide-eyed, and pulled into themselves. Many could only focus on the concrete. The elasticity of the mind was gone. Instead these Katrina victims often seemed to be in a "state of mindlessness," a term used by Boulanger to characterize the loss of symbolic function after massive trauma (p. 22). Some Katrina evacuees in the shelters, who had access to their emotional experiences, were helped by talking about them. It is important that those who need to talk have the opportunity to do so. A psychoanalytic approach to disaster relief factors in differences in individual functioning and allows for exploration when needed. I've seen non-analytic responders tell victims it is wrong or unhelpful to focus on feelings at the beginning. I consider this a misuse of psychological first aid guidelines and most importantly it doesn't recognize and accept the disaster victim as he is at that moment.

Over the last decade psychological first aid has gained prominence as the preferred psychosocial intervention for individuals who have suffered highly traumatic events (Vernberg et al., 2008). In the wake of 9/11 and catastrophic disasters such as Hurricane Katrina in the United States, and terrorist attacks and disasters worldwide, efforts have focused on establishing structured guidelines for providing psychological first aid to adults, children, and families. These include "Psychological First Aid: Field Operations Guide," developed jointly by the National Child Traumatic Stress Network and the National Center for Posttraumatic Stress Disorders (Brymer et al., 2006) and "Psychological First Aid: Guide for Field Workers" a collaboration among the World Health Organization (WHO), War Trauma Foundation, and World Vision International (World Health Organization, War Trauma Foundation and World Vision International, 2011).

While psychological first aid draws on psychoanalytic concepts (for example, recognition of insults to the self and an inability to process and recognize affect), psychoanalysis is seldom, if ever, mentioned in the literature. For instance, Bisson and Lewis's (2009) systematic review of psychological first aid failed to mention the work of psychoanalyst Martin Symonds. Symonds (1977), writing about victims of senseless violence, said: "The principles of psychological first-aid involve the recognition and sharing of what happened, concern and relief for the safety of the victim, and acceptance without reservation, challenge or question of the victim's behavior under severe stress. It can and should be done by parents and all helping personnel" (p. 3). Symonds's cogent conceptualization of psychological first aid predates current conceptualizations by decades. Three decades later the resemblance is plain: “The goals of this core action [of psychological first aid] are to respond to and initiate contacts in a nonintrusive, compassionate, and helpful manner … At a very basic level, exposure to highly traumatic events induces a sense of disbelief and disconnection from normal human experience” (Vernberg et al., 2008, p. 383).

Clinical vignettes

Applied to the evacuees in the Dallas shelters, these three trauma theories reveal a population grossly vulnerable to traumatic stress disorders. An African-American woman, “Clara,” told me her “ground zero” experience. She lived with her grown daughter and grandchildren. They had no way to evacuate. They sat out the hurricane with inadequate food, water, and medicine. Finally, they loaded the children on a mattress and fastened a rope to pull it. They waded into the reeking water that at times reached their shoulders. They moved past human and animal corpses. Clara was without her diabetic medication. Her faith in humanity faltered as she thought she might die. She willed herself to go on for her daughter and grandchildren. They were finally rescued and relief came in the form of a bus to Houston, TX and from there to Dallas, TX. That’s where I met “Clara.” For the victims of Hurricane Katrina, “ground zero” was the experience of living through the breakdown of the levees and the even worse breakdown of humankind to come to their aid in the following days. Clara and her family were situated in the “zone of sadness” closest to ground zero.

Clara was no stranger to trauma. Her personal history was marked with it, including the very worst of Hurricane Katrina. My job was to help this woman who had traveled through hell and now lived on the floor of an arena, assigned to a cot, without one possession from her past. I talked to Clara about the strength I saw in her. I said she had gumption. When help didn’t come she and her family took off to save themselves. She had clearly raised her daughter to do the same because that was exactly what her daughter had done as well. I said they looked to me like a family of strong women who had what it takes to overcome what life throws at them. I told her now she could rest. We would look after the children. She could shower, sleep, eat, and get her hair done. We’d get her diabetic medication. She was safe. She didn’t have to stay alert for the next bad thing to happen.

My goal was to recognize and highlight her resiliency while giving her permission to stand down from her hyper-vigilant position.

An eight-year-old child, "Eva," tried to attach herself to my hip whenever I was in the shelter. She arrived in Dallas without her mother, but was accompanied by her grandmother. With no knowledge of her mother's fate, Eva was terrified. Unlike Clara, neither Eva nor her grandmother were able to articulate a coherent story. Eva told me I looked like her mother, despite the difference in our races. I wanted to comfort this child, but knew it was not in her best interest to develop an attachment to me, as I would not be working in that shelter for long. I hugged her when I saw her and talked with her about how strong and brave she was even when she didn't feel that way inside. It was natural and normal to feel scared and worried, but good, smart people were working hard to find her momma. I talked with her grandmother about resources within the shelter to draw upon when Eva needed comfort and support.

As I stood with a duffel bag full of toys in the midst of 40 children, the shelter director said to me, "They're all traumatized. Help them." I picked out a five-year-old boy and asked the staff to get two other children the same age. With so many children I didn't have time for individual interaction. I grouped them by age in order to meet them at their developmental level. I sat down with three five-year-olds and discovered I could barely understand the speech patterns of these African-American children from New Orleans. The acoustics in the arena, originally designed for basketball games, were no help. I began with identifying feelings. I asked what a feeling is and one wide-eyed boy said, "Sad." When I asked what made him sad he replied, "When my momma beats me." I tried to assess as best I could in the limited time and space the meaning of his statement. I decided it was likely he told me about what made him sad before the hurricane and the horrible journey he'd been through because he had no way yet to conceptualize his "ground zero" experience and no words to describe it. He fell back on his more familiar experience of sadness, namely maternal beatings of some sort. I couldn't investigate it and I was aware of the cultural gulf between us. It was possible that his life prior to Katrina was so chaotic and abusive that the hurricane was just one of a series of bad things that happened to him. I had neither the time nor the means to find out for certain.

I realized I had arrived without a plan or an idea of what was most needed. I stepped back and observed both the children and the staff. This shelter's director had established a secure play area for children, separate from the floor of the arena, the main living area. Another area was established for babies and toddlers. Employees of the Dallas Parks and Recreation Department ran both areas. I asked the staff what questions they had and what they needed. We decided I would provide them with developmental guidelines for children's reactions to trauma and ways to identify signs of distress that might require a mental health professional. The most vulnerable children were those separated from adult relatives and we worked to identify and help those children. The preteen and teenage boys were particularly restless and needed a physical outlet. It was difficult to arrange taking the children outside, but we managed to establish some set times for the boys to go outside and play basketball. I quickly realized this particular shelter was attending well to the needs of its children.

I sat on a cot with a ten-year-old girl whose name I never knew. Soon other girls joined us. All of them had come to Dallas from the damaged New Orleans Superdome; a roof collapse resulted in a loss of utilities and abysmal conditions. The conditions created suffering and aroused fear. Rumors circulated about rapes and killings. The girls had not witnessed or experienced these atrocities, but they believed they had occurred. At that point it was impossible to know the accuracy of the reports. It was clear the rumors/reports terrified these young girls. One of them said to me "I heard it was white boys." From the beginning I was acutely aware that almost all the evacuees were African-American while most shelter workers were Caucasian. Disaster work from a psychoanalytic perspective involves understanding the cultural context and quickly recognizing underlying fears and suspicions. I thought this young girl was trying to say that black people weren't to blame. This wasn't therapy. I couldn't say, "You heard it was white boys?" with that question mark at the end of the sentence that every psychoanalyst knows how to do. I chose not to focus on what had happened in the Superdome. Instead, I focused on the here-and-now relationship between us. I said I was glad she had brought up race because I noticed that most of the folks from New Orleans were black and most of the folks in Dallas working in the shelters were white. I asked if things being divided up like that felt kind of weird to her. She replied that she didn't want "us" (the white people) to look down on them because they (the black people) "didn't have nuthin." I said I didn't want that either. I said it sometimes really hurts to need help. It hurts your pride. I said the white people helping out felt bad for her and the others because of all the bad stuff they had to go through, but we didn't look down on them. I said I was impressed by how strong she and the others were to get through all of it and I didn't know if I could have been that strong. I said I hoped my child could be as strong as she and the others in the shelter.

During this discussion I noticed adults nearby straining to listen. In a louder voice I said if there was anything anyone could tell me about what they might need that I, as a white outsider, wouldn't know, I hoped they would tell me. Immediately a woman said, "We need black hair products. We can't use your products." After that I experienced a palpable release of tension. I can't say tension left the room because we were in a cavernous space, which was actually an indoor parking lot of the Convention Center. People didn't have rooms. They had cots and they identified their cot location by a number on a concrete post. Disaster work is often piecemeal. The few people within earshot heard our exchange, but hundreds and thousands of others did not. I also tried to make sure black hair products were ordered and distributed. I understood hair products to be an actual resource.

That discussion led me to think these children needed transitional objects to help them cope. Most had arrived with only the clothes on their backs. The blankets we provided for the younger children seemed inadequate. I developed a plan to give the children black dolls and black action figures. I wanted them to have something to cling to that looked like them. The best way to accomplish this in the short time available was to ask Dallas churches to send out their parishioners to buy them. Hundreds were donated. The sight of the children hugging these toys that resembled themselves filled me with tears. I had not learned this intervention from a manual. Like many disaster responses it was born out of a frustration to make even the smallest difference in the lives of those who survived. It was, also, born from my psychoanalytic background that understands attachment, transitional objects, and insults to the sense of self.

Months after the disaster I was part of a team meeting with a group of counselors and administrators from a school district in a Dallas suburb. One administrator, in an exasperated tone, told the story of a parent who wouldn't let her alone. He came to her office frequently to check on his children and parked his beat-up car in a no-parking zone. Each visit he told her he had three spotless cars in New Orleans, a beautiful century-old home, and much more. The administrator, overwhelmed by this sudden influx of students from a different city and culture, saw the parent as bothersome, bragging, and entitled. I pointed out that her stress was interfering with what I was sure were her usual empathic capacities. I asked her to think about what it was like to be this parent in a strange place, losing all his worldly possessions, and left living off the donations of strangers. I suggested that he felt powerless, overwhelmed, and as though his sense of who he was as a man had been beaten into the ground as surely as his house had been torn down to the ground. I used this imagery purposefully. It worked. The administrator realized his bragging about his cars was a way for him to say: "I'm somebody. I'm not a nobody." This led to a rich discussion of the different ways that individuals respond to trauma and how to be helpful in the face of trauma and stress-related behaviors. My psychoanalytic approach allowed this discussion to take place. One non-analytic clinician on the team tried to apply the psychological first aid principle of "not exploring feelings" to interactions with evacuees months after the disaster occurred. She told the counselors to discourage such exploration. Alternatively, I helped the counselors think about being attuned to the psychological state of each person they encountered and to respond based on that attunement.

Organizational vignette

The psychiatry and psychology departments at the University of Texas Southwestern Medical Center established a psychiatric emergency room in the Red Cross shelter. The ER was an important resource for the many evacuees with pre-existing psychiatric disorders, but not for the majority of evacuees who were stressed, but didn't need psychiatric care. The departments established support groups called Psychological Aid Group Education (PAGE), which focused on "normalizing patients' experiences, educating patients about trauma responses, and promoting resiliency." The groups, planned three times a day, were largely unattended. Several factors contributed to this failure. The groups followed standard principles of psychological first aid, but the non-analytic clinicians who designed them lacked disaster experience. They didn't recognize a core principle of analytic disaster work: getting to know the disaster victims. They pathologized disaster victims by thinking of them as patients, a label rightly rejected by the evacuees. The groups needed a name that potential attendees could accept, such as "Support Group." Most importantly, the clinicians needed to meet with the evacuees where they lived, on their cots, eating meals, and standing in line for services. In a Red

Cross shelter, disaster victims are too traumatized and focused on survival to think of coming to a psychological support group. The heart of psychoanalytic mental health disaster relief is talking with the victims to provide them a sense of support and understanding. Such contact facilitates victims coming to support groups and without such contact they are unlikely to attend.

The largest Red Cross shelter, unlike my first shelter, had no provisions for children. Another clinician and I worked to establish a separate center for children where they could be cared for while their parents worked to get their lives back in order. Having seen what was done at the first shelter I thought I knew what to do. I was wrong. We never succeeded. We went to the shelter director, to the directors of the Psych ER, to the City of Dallas Crisis Intervention leader, to the Federal Emergency Management Agency (FEMA) and eventually to the CEO of the Dallas Red Cross Chapter. The CEO told us to select a child care group to run such a facility for children. When they tried to enter the shelter they were turned away at the door. This director had different priorities from those of the first shelter. This experience taught me where the power lies in a Red Cross shelter—with the director. Our time would have been far better spent establishing rapport and building a dialogue with the shelter director.

Conclusion

This chapter highlights the multiple and sequential traumas experienced by the Katrina victims who came to Dallas. Katrina barreled down on a New Orleans whose residents were often already acquainted with trauma. They were further traumatized by the hurricane and its aftermath: the conditions in New Orleans, particularly the conditions at the so-called shelters, the Superdome and the Convention Center, and by relocation to shelters in Dallas (often via Houston).

The shelters were closed after 15 days, when "Project Exodus," a collaboration between the city of Dallas and Dallas churches, provided apartments and hotel rooms for the evacuees. The churches provided all initial funding and FEMA eventually stepped up to the plate. On several occasions the victims were precipitously informed their housing would no longer be funded. They had no alternative place to live. Deadlines were announced, people panicked and finally deadlines were rescinded. Already living in a state of anxiety and tension, the evacuees were made more anxious and upset by the insensitivity of the government bureaucracy. These are just the large-scale traumas we know about. Were we to look closely at each individual life, I believe we would find many more insults to the self that add to the "pile of trauma" borne by the Katrina victims.

What kind of impact will the traumas of Hurricane Katrina have on its victims? The evacuees with whom I worked most closely were often from the poorest neighborhoods and had the hardest lives prior to Katrina, leaving them more prone to further traumatizations. The prevalence of mental illness is highest among socially and economically disadvantaged populations (Fryers, Melzer and Jenkins, 2003). A year following Hurricane Katrina, New Orleans residents who were disadvantaged and uneducated had higher rates of mental illness than those with more education and income (Sastry and VanLandingham, 2009).

Children, especially young children, are particularly vulnerable to trauma (Osofsky, 2011). Children who have faced previous trauma are more likely to develop symptoms of a stress disorder. Extensive exposure to the traumatic event, loss of a loved one, separation from a parental figure, previous trauma and negative changes in parental figures contribute, individually and collectively, to the development of stress disorders in children (McFarlane, 1987; Aisenberg and Mennen, 2000; Scheeringa and Zeanah, 2001; DeVoe et al., 2011). Thus, the children I encountered in the shelters are likely to develop stress disorders.

The psychoanalytic, attachment, and trauma literatures inform us that traumatized children are at risk of developing mental disorders in both childhood and adulthood. As Terr (1991) writes, "childhood psychic trauma leads to a number of mental changes that eventually account for some adult character problems, certain kinds of psychotic thinking, considerable violence, much dissociation, and extremes in passivity, self-mutilative episodes, and a variety of anxiety disturbances" (p. 11). A wide spectrum of traumatized children exhibit the following features: strongly visualized or otherwise repeatedly perceived memories, repetitive behaviors, trauma-specific fears, and changed attitudes about people, aspects of life, and the future (Terr, 1991). Traumatized children who have lost their sense of invincibility see the future as filled with dangers, pitfalls, and monsters (Lifton and Olsen, 1976). Not all Katrina children or even a majority will show these kinds of responses. But the mental health profession must focus on those who do.

The physical, emotional, and psychic havoc wrought by Katrina and its ugly aftermath left few unscathed, regardless of race, social class, or mental health functioning. Boulanger (2007) has documented the adult onset of trauma in individuals with no identified predispositions for post-traumatic stress reactions. Those with resources, however, are most likely to be able to rebuild their homes and their lives. Those without resources remain at risk in a city where mental health services had been cut by 75 percent before the hurricane hit. For those multiply disadvantaged, the years that followed the devastation have often been filled with continued loss and frustration. Our nation has never seen the level of devastation that Katrina brought to New Orleans and the Gulf Coast. While a city is being rebuilt, the people of the city, returned or scattered, will never be the same.

I encourage other psychoanalysts and psychoanalytic therapists to join me in mental health disaster relief work. We bring an important and unique perspective to this work. For example, when the girls talked about atrocities in the Superdome I looked beyond the content and attended to the dynamics of their fears or beliefs. By addressing the relationship between us, I acknowledged a relational dynamic (our racial differences) and brought it out in the open to be discussed. After that exchange, as well as others, I left the shelter inwardly thankful for my psychoanalytic training.

I was most successful when guided by my psychoanalytic perspective and least successful when I strayed from my dynamic roots. That same psychoanalytic orientation, however, helped me realize my errors. This first occurred when I entered the shelter and immediately accepted the director's appeal to help the 40 or so traumatized children. I was overwhelmed by the task. I failed to stop and ask what this feeling was telling me about myself and the situation. My initial intervention was ill-planned. When I regained my analytic footing, I realized I was acting out my desire to help and make contact with each child personally. My interventions were more to make me feel better about helping than actually to help in an attuned way to the needs of the children and the staff. Once I gained this insight I was able to help the staff find ways to be attuned to the needs of these traumatized, displaced children and help them begin to gain some sense of security.

My failed efforts to establish a child care center in the largest shelter is another example of losing my psychoanalytic grounding. I became overly determined to achieve my goal and I proceeded to plow through all possible sources to get my way. I forgot the importance of a therapeutic alliance. Had I remembered first and foremost to "pay attention to the relationship" (with the shelter director), the outcome may have been different. I still may have failed, but I might have deepened my understanding of the systemic resistances to providing services for children. As psychoanalytic clinicians we approach the challenges of disaster work with the benefit of looking for solutions in the content, the process, and the cultural context. Our depth approach enables us to use both self and other as we help victims of disaster turn into survivors. These skills differentiate us from other clinicians doing disaster work and equip us especially well for the task.

Note

1 Reprinted from *Psychoanalysis, Culture & Society, suppl. Special Issue: Psychoanalysis, Trauma, and Community* 18.2 (Jun 2013): 153–166 by permission of Palgrave Macmillan.

An earlier version of this chapter was presented at the annual meeting of the Division of Psychoanalysis, San Antonio, TX, 22–26 April, 2009 as part of the panel "Psychoanalysis in the Trenches: Perspectives on Trauma and Disaster."

References

Aisenberg, E. and Mennen, F. (2000) Children exposed to community violence: Issues for assessment and treatment. *Child and Adolescent Social Work Journal* 17 (5): 341–360.

Benight, C. (2012) Understanding human adaptation to traumatic stress exposure: Beyond the medical model. *Psychological Trauma, Theory, Research, Practice and Policy* 4 (1): 1–8.

Bisson, J. and Lewis, C. (2009) Systematic review of psychological first aid. Commissioned by the World Health Organization. http://mhpss.net/wp-content/uploads/group-documents/148/1321872322-PFASystematicReviewBissonCatrin.pdf, accessed August 8, 2012.

Boulanger, G. (2005) From voyeur to witness: Recapturing symbolic function after massive psychic trauma. *Psychoanalytic Psychology* 22 (1): 21–31.

Boulanger, G. (2007) *Wounded by Reality: Understanding and Treating Adult Onset Trauma*. New York: The Analytic Press.

Bowlby, J. (1969) *Attachment and Loss (Vol. 1), Attachment*. New York: Basic Books.

Brymer, M., Jacobs, A., Layne, C., Pynoos, R., Ruzek, J., Steinberg, A., Vernberg, E. and Watson, P. (2006) *Psychological First Aid: Field Operations Guide*, 2nd edn. Los Angeles: National Child Traumatic Stress Network and National Center for PTSD, www.nctsn.org and www.ncptsd.va.gov, accessed August 8, 2012.

Calera, T., Palma, L., Penayo, U. and Kullgren, G. (2001) Psychological impact of the Hurricane Mitch in Nicaragua in a one-year perspective. *Social Psychiatry and Psychiatric Epidemiology* 36 (3): 108–114.

Carlson, D. and Dallenberg, C. (2000) A conceptual framework for the impact of traumatic experiences. *Trauma, Violence and Abuse* 1 (1): 4–28.

DeVoe, E., Klein, T., Bannon, W. and Mirando-Julian, C. (2011) Young children in the aftermath of the World Trade Center attacks. *Psychological Trauma, Theory, Research, Practice and Policy* 3 (1): 1–7.

Freedy, J., Saladin, M., Kilpatrick, D., Resnick, H. and Saunders, B. (1994) Understanding acute psychological distress following natural disaster. *Journal of Traumatic Stress* 7 (2): 257–273.

Fryers, T., Melzer, D. and Jenkins, R. (2003) Social inequalities and the common mental disorders. *Social Psychiatry and Psychiatric Epidemiology* 38 (5): 229–237.

Hobfoll, S.E. (1989) Conservation of resources: A new attempt at conceptualizing stress. *American Psychologist* 44 (3): 513–524.

Hobfoll, S.E. (1991) Traumatic stress: A theory based on rapid loss of resources. *Anxiety Research* 4 (3): 187–189.

Hobfoll, S.E., Watson, P., Bell, C.C., Bryant, R.A., Brymer, M.J., Friedman, M.J., Friedman, M., Gersons, B.P., de Jong, J.T., Layne, C.M., Maguen, S., Neria, Y., Norwood, A.E., Pynoos, R.S., Reissman, D., Ruzek, J.I., Shalev, A.Y., Solomon, Z., Steinberg, A.M., Ursano, R.J. (2007) Five essential elements of immediate and mid-term mass trauma intervention: Empirical evidence. *Psychiatry* 70 (4): 283–315.

Kessler, R. (2000) Posttraumatic stress disorder: The burden to the individual and to society. *Journal of Clinical Psychiatry* 61 (5): 4–14.

Kolassa, I.-T., Verena, E., Eckart, C., Kolassa, S., Onyut, L. and Elbert, T. (2010) Spontaneous remission from PTSD depends on the number of traumatic event types experienced. *Psychological Trauma, Theory, Research, Practice and Policy* 2 (3): 169–174.

Leary, K. (2006) In the eye of the storm. *Psychoanalytic Quarterly* 75 (1): 345–363.

Lifton, J. and Olsen, E. (1976) The human meaning of total disaster. *Psychiatry* 39 (1): 1–18.

McFarlane, A. (1987) Posttraumatic phenomena in a longitudinal study of children following a disaster. *Journal of the American Academy of Child and Adolescent Psychiatry* 26 (5): 764–769.

Muesser, K., Trumbetta, S. Rosenberg, S., Vidaver, R., Goodman, L., Osher, F. and Auciello, P. (1998) Trauma and posttraumatic stress disorder in severe mental illness. *Journal of Consulting and Clinical Psychology* 66 (3): 493–499.

North, C., Kawasaki, A., Spitznagel, E. and Hong, B. (2004) The course of PTSD, major depression, substance abuse and somatization after a natural disaster. *Journal of Nervous and Mental Disease* 192 (12): 823–829.

Osofsky, J. (2011) Young children and disaster: Lessons learned from Hurricane Katrina about the impact of disasters and post disaster recovery: Clinical work with traumatized young children. In: J. Osofsky (ed.) *Clinical Work with Traumatized Young Children*. New York: Guilford Press, pp. 295–312.

Picou, S. and Marshall, B. (2007) Katrina as a paradigm-shift: Reflections on disaster research in the twenty-first century. In: D. Brunsma, D. Oversvelt and J.S. Picou (eds) *The Sociology of Katrina: Perspectives on a Modern Catastrophe*. Lanham: Rowman and Littlefield, pp. 1–20.

Sastry, N. and VanLandingham, M. (2009) One year later: Mental illness prevalence and disparities among New Orleans residents displaced by Hurricane Katrina. *American Journal of Public Health* 3 (3): 725–731.

Scheeringa, M. and Zeanah, C. (2001) A relational perspective on PTSD in early childhood. *Journal of Traumatic Stress* 14 (4): 799–815.

Scott, T. (2007) Multiple experiences and the development of posttraumatic stress disorder. *Journal of Interpersonal Violence* 22 (7): 932–938.

Slade, A. (2000) The development and organization of attachment: Implications for psychoanalysis. *Journal of the American Psychoanalytic Association* 48 (4): 1147–1174.

Strozier, C. (2002) The World Trade Center disaster and the apocalyptic. *Psychoanalytic Dialogues* 12 (3): 361–380.

Symonds, M. (1977) Victims of senseless violence. *Psychiatric Worldview* 1: 1–3.

Terr, L. (1991) Childhood traumas: An outline and overview. *American Journal of Psychiatry* 148 (1): 10–20.

Vernberg, E., Steinberg, A., Jacobs, A., Brymer, M., Watson, P., Osofsky, J., Layne, C., Pynoos, R. and Ruzek, R. (2008) Innovations in disaster mental health: Psychological first aid. *Professional Psychology: Research and Practice* 39 (4): 381–388.

World Health Organization, War Trauma Foundation and World Vision International. (2011) *Psychological First Aid: Guide for Field Workers*. Geneva: WHO.

Chapter 4

Some dark reality

A community develops skills to cope with shared trauma[1]

Ghislaine Boulanger

> We share some dark reality and we avoid the necessary inquiry into that reality ... A sense of togetherness and at the same time acute loneliness because our unique experiences are not being shared.
>
> (Hanoch Yerushalami, personal communication, 2008)[2]

Confronted with painful, sometimes unimaginably graphic details from survivors of violent or catastrophic events, many psychodynamic clinicians find themselves vicariously traumatized, feeling as if they have actually lived through the events they are hearing about. But when the clinician has survived the same or similar experiences as those who are seeking her professional counsel, the term vicarious no longer applies. Rather, the clinician is thrown into the looking glass world of shared trauma, where her own experiences, her reactions to them, her self-doubts, fears and terrors mirror her patients' own and are reflected back in ways that are deeply disturbing.

This was the dilemma facing local clinicians in New Orleans in the wake of Hurricane Katrina. At best, those who had evacuated shared with their patients exposure to images of collective death and vast suffering, a vision of their city disappearing under the flood waters; at worst, they had been among those left behind struggling to stay ahead of the flood. When they returned to the city, a post-apocalyptic world awaited clinicians and patients alike. The physical and social fabric of their lives had been destroyed.

Bollas (2009) points out that we do not usually develop a narrative about the dailyness of our material world; the visual, nameless forms that establish familiarity and consistency exist in a preverbal world of signs, senses, smells, affinities that constitute life in the maternal order. Another way of saying this is that as we grow beyond infancy, we continue to live in a holding environment that affords us the psychic energy to go on being while we conduct much of the rest of our lives in the symbolic order. How do mental health professionals continue to provide a holding environment for their patients when the larger maternal order has been catastrophically overturned?

In the weeks, months, and years after the storm many clinicians in New Orleans did continue to treat ongoing patients and take new referrals.[3] In this chapter I describe the different phases these clinicians passed through: from the immediate aftermath of the storm, to a crisis of confidence in their own work and their professional skills, to a new resolution that led to deeper connections to their patients. Simultaneously, I examine the underlying shifts in physical, therapeutic, and personal boundaries that are inevitable under conditions of shared trauma.[4]

Within days of the storm, even as the city was still under evacuation orders, some clinicians volunteered in programs providing psychological first aid and other interventions aimed at fostering resilience among first responders and their families. Others, many in private practice, felt a pressing need to make contact with patients who had not already reached out to them. They were determined to keep working, to re-establish their professional identity and familiar routines in a chaotic and unpredictable world.

But the work was not familiar; some obvious boundaries had been lost, others blurred. For many, the physical surround in which their work took place was no longer available; they were practicing in makeshift offices, sometimes in different cities; some conducted telephone sessions for the first time. As they established new schedules in different locations, the usual therapeutic stance was abandoned and other boundaries called into question. Patients asked direct questions—"Where did you evacuate to?" "Did you have much damage?" "Is everyone OK?" Many psychodynamic clinicians felt it was "inhuman" not to address these concerns, but, in breaking with their normal practice, they feared they were being unprofessional. During that first year one clinician confided, "We couldn't get shit done, but just staying the course, being there, providing continuity felt important."

Within weeks, sometimes months, doing treatment was no longer serving as a manic defense against the chronic sense of vulnerability to which

Katrina had given rise. Clinicians could no longer keep up the pretense that it was business as usual. On a manifest level they were struggling with doubts about the quality of their work. They asked themselves, "Am I doing this right or am I making it worse?" "She knows I had to move; what else can I let her know?" "Do I want her to know?" "What if she's doing better than me?" "As a therapist I'm supposed to be OK but am I OK? Am I recovering from the storm or just pretending?" "What am I bringing into treatment sessions from my own life?" "Does anyone else feel this way?"

Unconsciously trauma works insidiously to throw less obvious but long established boundaries into question. What had felt like small transgressions were followed by others that caused greater concern. Much of the time, these boundaries are taken for granted, but in the wake of a massive trauma, the line between reality and fantasy has been breached. This is what Fonagy, Gergely, Jurist and Target (2002) describe as psychic *equivalence*, signifying that the internal world and the external world have merged. In the state of psychic equivalence, the boundaries between self and other, between inner and outer, between past, present and future, and between private and public blur. Personal and professional lives collide, Floyd writes her account of the treatments she was doing after the storm: "I was beginning to recognize, in a visceral way, the intersection between the 'stories' I was hearing and the story I was living" (Boulanger, Floyd, Nathan, Poitevant and Pool, 2013, p. 20).

Following a psychic trauma, whether listening closely to details or emerging from the experience itself, clinicians frequently find that the internal space necessary to think clearly, to reflect, to hold onto the distinction between their own internal experiences and their patients' has been compromised. "We are deskilled by trauma," Saakvitne (2002) wrote after the destruction of the Twin Towers. Under these circumstances, thinking symbolically, giving meaning to experience is next to impossible. One experienced analyst hinted at the collapse of an additional unseen boundary in expressing her frustration about her post-Katrina work: "It took a while to start thinking about Katrina in psychological terms. I couldn't think about it. I couldn't do it. I didn't do it because I couldn't do it." Psychodynamic clinicians are taught to pay attention to underlying meanings, but in post-Katrina New Orleans's underlying meanings proved elusive or felt contrived. In effect, the distinction between psychic reality and external reality had collapsed. Instead of interpreting, clinicians had to listen, sometimes repeatedly, to their patients' horrifying narratives and painful re-entry experiences, or encourage them to explore them, or ignore them—at their peril.

In closely following a trauma narrative, containing another's terror can begin to reverse the experience of psychic equivalence starting to differentiate past and present, outside and inside, reality and fantasy, self and other. But in undertaking this task, the clinicians were contending with their own reluctance to be exposed and re-exposed to accounts that were painfully familiar, concerned that they themselves had not made a good enough recovery from the storm. Months and often years later, finding patients who still needed help with the intrusive memories of the storm and its aftermath and despair about their living conditions, clinicians still found themselves reluctant to engage these narratives, consciously, and sometimes unconsciously, fearing that in the critical moment they would not be up to the task of containing their patients' unmentalized experiences, but would instead be overwhelmed by their own memories, memories that would not stay in the past, and with ongoing disbelief about their own experiences. This is the "dark reality" to which Yerushalami (2008) refers in the epigraph to this chapter; the recognition that personal lives, professional lives, and patients' lives cannot be kept separate after a shared trauma.

The fundamental premise of the treatment relationship is that it is asymmetrical (Aron, 1996). Even among those who believe in the inevitable mutuality of a two-person treatment, it is understood that certain responsibilities, functions, and power are accorded to those who assume the role of therapist. This is the basis of the working alliance. But that working alliance is challenged by shared trauma. The dark reality casts a pall on relationships with colleagues; often the clinician's self-doubt and shame lead to a reluctance to share their concern with other professionals and a profound sense of isolation.

At first clinicians dreaded this suddenly symmetrical relationship; it represented a loss of a familiar professional identity, a loss of omnipotence leading to humiliation and confusion. Sometimes, but rarely, psychoanalysts refused to answer straightforward questions, interpreting them instead, thereby alienating their patients. In the end, however, most local mental health professionals who lived through Hurricane Katrina and committed to rebuilding their personal and professional lives in New Orleans came to understand that weathering the vicissitudes of shared trauma, acknowledging their own dissociative tendencies, and following closely their patients' evolving narratives, subtly changed the ways in which they practiced. Those who went into the dark reality with their patients found unexpected rewards. Even those who had not previously practiced intersubjectively came to recognize considerable benefits in the freedom that the brief interlude of symmetry afforded them. What had been an unwelcome intrusion turned into a new understanding about how to be available to patients emotionally, how to resonate to loss and horror in their own and other people's lives. Pool (2013) describes "a newfound understanding of the human factor." In Boulanger et al. (2013), Floyd wrote of the lasting benefit of having shared the intimate experience of trauma with so many people, "In the simplest terms, it's enhanced my capacity to 'get' it, it's so rich … Even when we aren't dealing with the storm, I understand what people have gone through in a different way, it's not just empathy; here's a new kind of understanding, recognition of what people are saying" (p. 22).

Notes

1 I am grateful to Kathy Nathan, Ph.D., of the New Orleans Birmingham Psychoanalytic Center who recognized the need for this study and Shirlee Taylor, Ph.D., of the Far Fund for underwriting the project on which this report is based. For in-depth discussion of this topic see Boulanger, Floyd, Nathan, Poitevant and Pool, 2013, and Boulanger, 2013, and a website designed for clinicians finding themselves in similar circumstances: http://www.therapistspostdisaster.com/index.html, accessed July 6, 2016.

2 This personal communication is reprinted in this chapter with the permission of Hanoch Yerushalami.

3 It is estimated that, depending on their discipline and location, between 35 percent and 85 percent of mental health professionals in the greater New Orleans area relocated after the storm (Faust, Black, Abrahams, Warner and Bellando, 2008).

4 Sampson, a psychotherapist in New Zealand, reported an identical pattern of responses among 15 colleagues she formally interviewed in the months and years following four major earthquakes in Christchurch (personal communications, 2013, 2014).

References

Aron, L. (1996). *A Meeting of Minds: Mutuality in Psychoanalysis*. Hillsdale, NJ: The Analytic Press.

Bollas, C. (2009). *The Evocative Object World*. London, New York: Routledge.

Boulanger, G. (2013). Fearful Symmetry: Shared Trauma in New Orleans after Hurricane Katrina. *Psychoanalytic Dialogues*, 23(1): 31–44.

Boulanger, G., Floyd, L., Nathan., Poitevant, D. and Pool, E. (2013). Reports from the Front: The Effects of Hurricane Katrina on Mental Health Professionals in New Orleans. *Psychoanalytic Dialogues*, 23(1): 15–30.

Faust, D., Black, F., Abrahams, J., Warner, M. and Bellando, B. (2008). After the Storm: Katrina's Impact on Psychological Practice in New Orleans. *Professional Psychology: Research and Practice*, 39(1): 1–6.

Fonagy, P., Gergely, G., Jurist, E. and Target, M. (Eds) (2002). *Affect Regulation, Mentalization, and the Development of the Self.* New York: Other Press.

Saakvitne, K. (2002). Shared Trauma: The Therapist's Increased Vulnerability. *Psychoanalytic Dialogues*, 12: 443–449.

Chapter 5

Psychoanalysis in and out of the office[1]

Neil Altman

Introduction

Most analysts around the world have come to take for granted that psychoanalysis is an office-based practice. I will suggest that this location for psychoanalysis is an historical artifact—that, in fact, psychoanalysis can be practiced in the community, out of the office, and needs to be so practiced if it is to survive with much social relevance. With respect to trauma, in particular, human societies contain many individuals who have suffered, and are suffering, a variety of traumata, including ongoing traumatizing circumstances such as extreme material poverty, brutal discrimination, war, untreated and unnecessary illness and death. Most such people will never show up in a psychoanalyst's private office. If we, as analysts, insist that our work can take place only in the professional office, we will, in effect, be failing to address the most urgent forms of suffering around us. Psychoanalysis, I suggest, is about the engagement of suffering, including the inevitable inclination to avoid suffering. We cannot succeed as psychoanalysts if we fail to examine how and why we insulate ourselves from so much suffering.

Some might suggest that analysts can and should go out of their offices to reach a broader range of people, but that such work is not psychoanalysis, but rather, some form of psychotherapy or social work. I maintain, however, that psychoanalysis is defined by a focus on unconscious processes, especially transference/countertransference processes. By this definition, the professional field of psychoanalysis often fails to make an essential contribution to those who work in community-based settings. The field, in turn, is deprived to an extent of what might be learned from an expanded engagement with the world. Both psychoanalysts and community-based mental health workers can be greatly enriched by an expanded interaction.

How did psychoanalysis come to be thought of by many as *necessarily* office-based? I posit that the office context, the traditional frame thought to be necessary, and the Northern European/North American cultural context, are all of a piece. The traditional frame, as we know, emphasized reserve, non-gratification of the patient's wishes, and, to the extent that it was possible, anonymity. Standardizing the context seemed to promote these conditions. This standardization seems unfeasible once one leaves the office and enters the patient's world. The idea of the silent, reserved analyst best fits with a Northern European cultural context that values independence and tolerance for frustration. When there is a cultural fit, patients will most likely buy in, so to speak, to the values and theory underwriting the psychoanalytic method, according to which psychopathology is located within the individual patient's mind, knowable by the analyst in an objective way and from a detached perspective.

Incidentally, or not so incidentally, the office location allows the analyst to be on his or her own turf, more or less in control of the context, without needing to take the time and expense to travel. These benefits to the analyst and demands on the analysand are rarely, if ever, an object of analytic discussion. The fact that the analyst does not get to know by acquaintance the people inhabiting the patient's world, nor the material conditions of the patient's life, is also generally not discussed or even acknowledged to be the case, much less of significance in the analytic work itself.

Relational developments in psychoanalysis have opened up the analytically relevant context to include the larger social field, the patient–analyst dyad, the social location of analyst and analysand and the method itself, in terms of culture, value systems, and various forms of privilege and power. Once the psychoanalytic method is seen as culturally located, it becomes conceivable to consider and adopt various other frames. The office location is not imperative when standardization of the context, or objectivity aside from subjectivity, is not thought to be necessary, or even possible. When ego strength or analyzability is not defined in terms of a cultural fit between the analysand, the analyst, and the analytic method, the analyst can begin to think in terms of a cultural negotiation in which the analyst and the method itself must be flexible in order to be available to the analysand, and in which the analysand must reach out as well to meet the analyst. In certain cases, if any contact is to be made, and analytic work to occur, the analyst must reach out physically by going into the community.

Meanwhile, the broader clinical context has changed, at least in the United States (US), with more public mental health work going on out of the office or clinic. In the US, the Community Mental Health Act (1963) envisioned that community-based clinics and outreach programs would reduce the need for hospitalization. In the period between the 1970s and the present, community-based clinics have been replaced by the expectation that intensive case managers would be assigned to "at-risk" people and families for round-the-clock crisis management and follow-up to ensure treatment compliance. For the most part, states and cities have failed adequately to fund community-based mental health services; many people who would otherwise have been treated in community-based mental health systems have ended up in prison (Kupers, 1999).

Attunement to countertransference, or one's own subjective and emotional state, in out-of-office work

There are various programs designed to reach out to groups of people who are not familiar or comfortable with traditional forms of therapy and who must be met where they live if they are to be engaged at all. For example, the West Coast Children's Clinic in Oakland, California, has received funding from the government at various levels for therapeutic work with foster children and their families in their communities. The rate of payment is intended to compensate for time spent traveling to client's homes, sometimes over an hour each way.

In my view, working with people in their homes, often in the middle of a crisis, makes a psychoanalytic perspective even more useful, not to say necessary, than it is in the office. Imagine walking into a middle-of-the-night crisis in someone's home without the finely honed familiarity with your own feelings and subjective state, and the feelings and subjectivity of others, that the study of transference and countertransference often produces. Consider, for example, the following description of a clinician's experience as he approaches a client's home for a therapeutic visit:

> As I drive up to the house, I have the sense that I am an intruder, that those I am visiting are ambivalent at best about my coming into their home.

I park a couple of spots away from the house, wondering if my client will be walking down the street from her bus stop, past my car. What should I be doing as she walks past? I think of her foster mother, who is fed up with her and accuses me of being too soft on her because I don't demand information out of her the way she does. I get out of my car, sleepy from the drive, my eyes having been glued to the road for over an hour.

I walk across the street, nervous about what to address in today's session. If I decide to introduce something, it is certain to lead to bouts of silence. I always feel a bit silly walking with my play/art kit, which is translucent. I walk over the grass, since the car is blocking the driveway. I never thought to ask if it's OK that I walk on the grass. Maybe I should have.

As I approach the door, I become a therapist, and for a moment I realize that working in my client's home is a privilege. This thought quickly dissipates and I continue to feel me becoming the therapist. This therapist is me, only not. It's me, but only certain parts of me. The other parts of me push and yell to be seen, but I beat them back with conscience and pride. I am sort of a therapist/supervisor with her foster mother, so I let out more parts with her, but it's still a battle, albeit in the good war. I want to scream at her that she needs to meet with me and ease up on her expectations, and please tell your foster child that you love her, and oh, be nice to me while you're at it—but that wouldn't be therapeutic. I become a receptor of information. Moving slowly, taking everything in. Planning my next move. There is no such thing as routine or automatic.

There is a moment when I begin to panic. I wonder about myself, how others—my clients—see me, and how I see others. Questions begin to take over my mind. Am I smart enough? Cultured enough? Steeped in theory enough? Trained enough? Experienced enough? Wise enough? Thoughtful enough? Understand my role enough? Did I ask enough questions? Listen enough? Engage enough? Empathize enough? Am I patient enough? Assertive enough? Direct enough? Compassionate enough? Tough enough? Am I brown enough? Gay enough? Straight enough? Female enough? Oppressed enough? Am I spiritual enough? Open-minded enough? Aware enough? Sensitive enough? Conscious enough? Affirming enough? Humble enough? Respectful enough? Human enough? Can my clients see themselves in me? And what of me will I see in them?

The apartment is two stories but small and dark. A child opens the door, and I am assaulted by loud gospel music, screaming children, barking dogs, a hissing cat, and the smell of fried chicken. There are several young children running and playing in a living room that is smaller than one of our (clinic) playrooms. The children run up to me, pull at my coat, attempt to go through my kit, and demand to know why I am there. Where could we meet? Well, right there in that room filled with children, dogs, and music. Huh, I think. This will challenge my ability to maintain confidentiality. And once again, I am thrown into a crazy situation where boundaries are forced to stretch and I with them.

(previously quoted in Altman, 2009, pp. 215–216)

If it's out of the office, is it really psychoanalysis?

A traditional analyst might easily conclude that the situation described above is unfit for psychoanalytic work. But why? Because this is an unstandardized situation, any observations made of the patient in a one-person model are bound to be context-dependent. The analyst/therapist, off his/her familiar turf, is continually destabilized by unpredictable events. There is no calm center from which to make objective observations or even to reflect with any sort of leisure on what is transpiring. Interpretations seem out of the question. Keeping one's head above water seems the order of the day.

On the other hand, there are disadvantages, from an analytic point of view, to the office-based situation, of which we might not be aware since we take it for granted as the "standard." The patient is off his or her familiar turf, especially if he or she lives in the sort of environment described above. Yes, the analyst may be in control of the office-based situation, but that control may be an artifact of the office, with the sense of destabilization displaced onto the analysand. The sense that the patient can be objectively observed in the office may be largely illusory since the patient is in a unique situation, one he or she only encounters in real life when dealing with a functionary who has control over the patient, a control represented by the office—the functionary's turf. The analyst, as a person, can hide in the office. Again, vulnerability and destabilization are displaced onto the patient. The real conditions of the patient's life remain unknown to the analyst. How are lessons learned in the therapy supposed to be transferred into the patient's real life?

Of course, patients who inhabit offices on a regular basis, who feel at home there, are less likely to feel destabilized in the standard office-based situation. And that is precisely the point. The upper-socio-economic-class, culturally Northern European patient is most comfortable in the analytic office, while the analyst is least at home in the home environment of the lower-socio-economic-class patient, especially when these patients belong culturally to the nations of the economically developing world. If we hope to engage such patients, it may be necessary to leave the comfort of our offices and engage people where they live or elsewhere in the communities where they live, work, or seek services. If we are unwilling to do so, we perpetuate the insularity and elitism of psychoanalysis, something we can ill afford to do at this moment in history.

Let us assume for the moment that the office serves the function of standardizing the psychoanalytic situation to some extent, while reducing extraneous stimulation to a minimum. If psychoanalysis is defined by its focus on transference/countertransference and the unconscious, do we not need psychoanalysis all the more when we leave our offices and engage our patients in the less predictable and controllable environments in the community? The clinician quoted above shows an attunement to, and ability to articulate, his moment-to-moment experience as he approaches his client's home. Without such attunement, fostered by a psychoanalytic focus on inner experience and anxiety, he might have been either overwhelmed or shut down by the experience. In neither case would he have been well positioned to respond sensitively to the experience of his clients as he enters their world.

Psychoanalytic experiences in India

I

In India this past summer, my colleagues and I at Ambedkar University of Delhi approached the task of training students to work in community-based non-governmental organizations (NGOs) with a psychoanalytic perspective. In India, opportunities for private practice are limited, so the career paths of psychoanalytic students will take them into NGOs where they might be part of a community of runaway children picked up in train stations, or students in an after-school program, to take just two examples. In such contexts, these clinicians will not be sitting in offices receiving patients who are motivated to come to their door; instead they will become part of the community, mixing with people where they live and study, finding opportunities to engage anxieties and defenses as they emerge in real life. We began by asking the students and ourselves to go into our own communities where we live, and engage in a conversation with someone across social class lines, someone with whom we would not normally engage in a personal way. In the classroom, these conversations would then be discussed with an eye to the emotional currents activated within them on conscious and unconscious levels, as well as the therapeutic potential within them. Here are some examples of what students reported.

One woman in her early twenties reported that she got into a rickshaw for a short trip. The driver was a man in his mid-forties. "Rickshaw drivers often talk to me, so I thought this would be a good opportunity for me to have a conversation," reported this open-faced young woman. As the rickshaw moved along in fits and starts in the heavy traffic of Delhi, the driver would turn around when there was a short stop to say something to his passenger. At the first stop, he said, "I have a son and a daughter and a computer." The student said nothing. At the next stop he said: "And I found my son watching one of 'those movies' on the computer." Again, the student said nothing and just listened. At the next opportunity, the driver said, "I guess he's getting to the age where he's having 'those desires'." And then, "I guess my daughter is having those desires, too," to which the student said, "Maybe so." At the next stop he said, "I have those desires," and then a question: "Do you have those desires?" To which she responded, "Not yet." And then she added, "Not since my mother died two years ago." Nearing their destination, the driver then said, "My wife and I didn't know anything about sex when we got married, but we've learned that sex is a very important part of a marriage." At which point, the destination reached, the conversation was over.

In the discussion of this conversation, another student asked what was on everyone's mind: "Were you scared?" To which the student replied, "At one point I wondered if I *should* be scared, but actually I wasn't."

My own conclusion is that this conversation was a kind of therapy session. The driver, finding a receptive listener, brought a problem: how to deal with his son's emerging sexuality in the age of the Internet. He found a daughter-type person who set limits ("not yet," she said about her own desires) while opening herself up in a personal way about the death of her mother and its impact on her own sexuality. With this frame in place, he could have a safe and straightforward conversation with her about sex, an experience that presumably will facilitate his ability to have a discussion with his children.

II

Another student reported that she had always wanted to talk with the woman who presses clothes in the building where the student lives. Awkwardly, she approached the "presswali" (as a woman who presses clothes is called in Hindi) and asked, "How many children do you have?" The presswali responded, "I have some children." The student inquired, "*Some* children?" The presswali replied: "During the day the men beat us, and at night they take us." The student, dumbfounded, did not know what to say, and the conversation ended.

In this case, the student, picking up on the unusual locution "some children" simply inquired about it in her own empathic tone of voice. The presswali responded with a dramatic opening up of the brutal conditions of her life and the fact that, her children having been forced on her, she did not differentiate them as individuals who could be counted, or who counted. It is also notable that she spoke of "we"—women or abused women, there was no distinction. The student, unprepared for the level of suffering opened up by her simple question, could not, for the moment, take it in.

In the discussion, we pondered the question of how the student might have followed up, or might still follow up. I raised the possibility that the presswali may have been saying, in effect, "You present yourself as wanting to know about my life. Well, let's get to the heart of the matter and see if you *really* want to know about my life." For the moment, the answer was "yes and no." Understanding the conversation this way raises questions and concerns about the whole project of trying to engage people whose lives are full of extreme suffering. Do we really want to know about it?

Asking this question illuminates the nature of the resistance to engaging people at the social margins, people impacted by material poverty, social exclusion, exploitation, and more than their share of disease and death. These are the people who contain the suffering that more materially privileged people try to avoid and segregate into a marginal place, socially and psychically, in their/our pursuit of an illusory safety, security, and invulnerability. We, the privileged students and practitioners of psychoanalysis, might say that we want to engage suffering, but the presswali isn't convinced. Yet, she opens up her life to the student; there is an invitation, along with a challenge, to enter.

In my view, the student didn't need to say anything beyond the point at which words stopped. Help and reassurance are beside the point, and not possible at that moment. All that is possible is to realize that in many ways one indeed does not want to know about the presswali's suffering and the way we "helping professionals" participate in, and are shaped by, an inequitable and exploitative society that dumps suffering on this woman and the socially marginal group, the "we" to whom she refers. That would be the first step toward opening up to an authentic desire to engage this woman's life. With her invitation and challenge, perhaps the presswali concisely "interprets" the psychological situation between herself and the student. In a similar way, all our patients, if we are listening, often interpret our countertransference resistances to knowing them and their suffering. Perhaps we should all be listening to the presswali as we seek to understand how it is that we, as a field and as individuals, avoid those at the social margins, and what is entailed in turning that around.

III

This last summer I spent some time visiting NGOs, all of which are in the community and many of which are in themselves communities. One such NGO is Salaam Baalak Trust (SBT), founded by the filmmaker Mira Nair, who made the movie *Salaam Bombay*. The film was about runaway children who live in the Bombay train station; the NGO has offices in train stations all over India, where workers, often themselves former runaway children, go onto the platforms each day to identify, and offer services to, children who have fled their homes for one reason or another. After an assessment, some children are returned to their homes, while others are offered a place to live and attend school in one of the residences run by SBT. One day, with a colleague who was planning to work at SBT, I attended a "City Walk"—a tour of the neighborhood around the Delhi train station conducted by former runaway children, now young adults, who described life in the train station in general, as well as their own personal experiences.

Our tour guide, a young man named Kumar, explained that he had run away from home in Bombay at the age of nine years after his older brother left home, leaving him the only child with his mother and alcoholic, abusive father. He got on a train, ending up in Patna, where he lived in an NGO's residence for some time, until he ran away from that residence and ended up in Delhi. He recounted that children who lived in the train station subsisted by picking pockets and selling tap water as bottled water. He said they commonly got addicted to sniffing white-out, sold and used marijuana and heroin, and got sexually exploited. Girls often got raped and/or lured or abducted to work as prostitutes. Nonetheless, he said, it took months or years to convince children to give up what they perceived as the freedom of life in the train station to come to SBT's residence nearby.

At one moment, Kumar and I were standing off to the side of the main group. After explaining how he had run away from home, he said, "I have never given up my childhood dream: I want to be a train driver." I blurted out: "I want to be a train driver too!" There followed a discussion of how one becomes a train driver in India. It sounded like a laborious and uncertain process, with success quite a long shot. In response to his question as to where my colleague and I were from, I said we were from New York. "Who discovered America?" he asked. Guessing that this question was intended to expose any arrogant, ignorant, colonialist tendencies, I said (proudly, I must admit), "No one knows!" To which he said, "Right!" "What year did Columbus arrive?" he asked. My colleague playfully responded, "In fourteen hundred and ninety two, Columbus sailed the ocean blue," as Kumar joined in. As we walked along, he said that Barack Obama was supposed to have come on a City Walk, but the Walk had been cancelled because his security detail was not convinced he could be protected. We laughed, looking at the milling crowds of people in the street, the people on nearby rooftops hanging clothes or leaning out of windows, at the people on the sidewalk, sometimes engaging in conversation with each other or with passersby. Kumar asked: "What is the difference between Democrats and Republicans?" I responded that each was like a certain Indian political party. We all agreed that we were more like Democrats and Congress Party members, less like Republicans or the Hindu nationalist party, the BJP.

Later, as I thought about how one would function with a psychoanalytic sensibility in an NGO community, I wondered if one could psychoanalytically consider Kumar's comment that he wanted to be a train driver. At the time, I unreflectively (on a conscious level) joined him: I wanted to be a train driver too. In that way, I was keeping a childhood dream of my own alive, and joining him in the way that was at hand. Later, when the pathway to the unconscious opened for me, I thought that he was saying, in effect, that he wanted to take control of his life. If I had been functioning as a psychoanalyst at that moment, would I have "done" something with this remark?

The traditional psychoanalytic thing would have been to "interpret" it: i.e. to say something on a conscious level, like: "You want to take control of your life." To me this seems clunky and contrived.

If I had been oriented to processing the interaction psychoanalytically, would I have made my comment about wanting to be a train driver too? Perhaps. I would have been interested in seeing where things went when we spoke "unconscious to unconscious." I also suspect I would have been thinking about what must already have happened for him to open up this unconscious piece to me. Did he routinely tell people about this ongoing childhood wish when he conducted city tours?

Going a step further, I asked myself: what *was* I saying when I told him that I also wanted to be a train driver? It seems to me that in my case my expressed wish had to do with the power behind me, the train, the engine, the people in the train. In traditional psychoanalytic terms, the appeal is phallic. I don't think that was the issue for Kumar, or if it was, only in part. I too wanted to be in control of my life, of course, so there was some overlap. But then I thought of another fantasy of mine: I love riding in trains so much because it is like being pulled in a baby stroller. I envy children I see riding in strollers, their eyelids drooping as they surrender to sleep and someone else takes on the burden of pushing.

Later, I shared some of these reflections with some of my university colleagues. One of them remembered a dream I had had the last time I was in Delhi, a year earlier. I had mentioned this dream in a class I was teaching. As I remembered it, I was in a train and the driver was sitting up front in an open compartment. I was worried that he would be exposed to unruly passengers, but no disorder broke out. The train reached the end of the line, pulling up smoothly to a stop. The driver got out, went up the steps of an out-of-service escalator, and disappeared into a crowd of people. I am not sure I fully remember what I made of the dream at the time. I think I had some thoughts about finishing that visit to India, about expecting some sort of danger, about being exposed, about finding that things weren't as worrisome as I had thought they might be, about the unknown future after leaving Delhi that year. I am now struck that I was neither a passenger nor the driver in this dream; the dreamer was an observer.

Having remembered this dream with the assistance of my colleague and his associations, I then had an idea as to what I would do if I were working as an analyst at SBT and Kumar told me his "dream" (!) from childhood. I would either ask him about his dreams, or tell him my dream. From that point, this analytic driver disappears into the crowd, and I cannot see what happens next.

Later, reading this account to another colleague, I noticed that I said Kumar was "conducting" a city tour, so we had an immediate context for his remark. I was the passenger and he was the conductor, if not the driver. So he was fulfilling his childhood dream already, and I was a passenger whose job it was to be driven. (At first I wrote, "let myself be driven"—as if I were in control even as the passenger!).

Is psychoanalysis defined by where it takes place?

I suggest that one can think of psychoanalysis as defined by a particular frame, or aspect of the frame, such as the professional office, or the couch, the frequency and length of sessions, and so on. One can think of psychoanalysis as defined by a method, for example, free association and interpretation, which requires a particular frame such as the analytic couch, the recumbent posture or the out-of-sight analyst. One can also think of psychoanalysis as applicable to *any* framework or method, such as the community-based settings I have referred to, and others. If community-based settings, along with the people who will only be reached in such settings, are ruled out for psychoanalytic work, both psychoanalysis and community-based work will be deprived of a potentially rich interaction. Community-based workers can benefit from the finely attuned attention to feelings, subjective states, and the transference/countertransference interaction that have been developed in psychoanalysis. As I have suggested, enhanced awareness of the flow of feelings and anxieties is, if anything, more essential in negotiating the complex environments found out of the office, as essential as this awareness is to in-office work. Further, I believe that psychoanalysis, too, can be the beneficiary of an essential spur to growth and development if it engages the kind of suffering found mostly out of the office.

Throughout the history of psychoanalysis the field has, for the most part, evolved and progressed by taking on problems and patient populations previously ruled out as unsuitable for analytic work. I am suggesting here that there are psychoanalytically informed ways of addressing the kinds of acute and chronic trauma encountered under conditions of extreme material poverty in India and elsewhere. This kind of rethinking requires a high level of rigor and faithfulness to what is essentially psychoanalytic. To do so, we must be open to radically rethinking the frame, including the location and nature of the contact. If we can be open to taking psychoanalysis out into the world in this way, we will expand the forms of suffering we are prepared to address; we will enrich our field while liberating ourselves from our attachment to a framework that is, like all frameworks, an historical artifact. The flexibility and cultural sensitivity thus acquired will, in turn, feed back into our clinical work with *all* patients.

I consider the experiences reported here to be clinical experiences in the full sense of the word. Certainly, they were processed with the students at the university with a clinical psychoanalytic sensibility and perspective in mind, and with an eye toward developing a method of using spontaneous interactions in the service of the expansion of consciousness and mentalization of chronic trauma. Main and Hesse (1990) and Coates (1998) have suggested that the traumatized parent's ability to mentalize is a protective factor against the intergenerational transmission of trauma to the next generation. The parent's ability to mentalize allows for the development of mentalization in the child, thus freeing the child from the implantation of "alien introjects" (Fonagy et al., 2002) that perpetuate the reliving of trauma. We at Ambedkar University of Delhi seek to develop a method for enhancing mentalization in ourselves and those with whom we work in the midst of chronic trauma and extreme suffering in communities where it is no small matter to tolerate and process experience.

Note

1 Reprinted from *Psychoanalysis, Culture & Society, suppl. Special Issue: Psychoanalysis, Trauma, and Community* 18.2 (Jun 2013): 128–139 by permission of Palgrave Macmillan.

References

Altman, N. (2009) *The Analyst in the Inner City: Race, Class, and Culture through a Psychoanalytic Lens*, 2nd edn. London and New York: Routledge.

Coates, S. (1998) Having a mind of one's own and holding the other in mind: Commentary on paper by Peter Fonagy and Mary Target. *Psychoanalytic Dialogues* 8 (1): 115–148.

Fonagy, P., Gergely, G., Jurist, E.L. and Target, M. (2002) *Affect Regulation, Mentalization, and the Development of the Self*. New York: Other Press.

Kupers, T. (1999) *Prison Madness: The Mental Health Crisis Behind Bars and What We Can Do About It*. San Francisco: Jossey-Bass.

Main, M. and Hesse, E. (1990) Parents' unresolved traumatic experiences are related to infant disorganized status: Is frightened and/or frightening parental behavior the linking mechanism? In: M.T. Greenberg, D. Cicchetti and E.M. Cummings (eds) *Attachment in the Preschool Years: Theory, Research, and Intervention*. Chicago: University of Chicago Press: 161–182.

Part III

Facilitating collective mourning

Chapter 6

Intervention strategies for addressing collective trauma

Healing communities ravaged by racial strife[1]

Ricardo C. Ainslie

Introduction

Psychoanalysis is a robust collection of concepts whose utility beyond the consulting room has yet to be fully understood or exploited. In the present contribution I describe three interrelated, psychoanalytically informed interventions. The interventions were part of a project in a Texas community where conflict-laden residues of the Jim Crow era continued to affect race relations. The first intervention (the creation of a space within which Jim Crow- and Civil Rights era narratives could be spoken and explored) and the second intervention (the creation of a documentary film) were closely linked because they were part of a process in which interviews gave testimony about a decisive, transformational experience. The third intervention created a public event where that which had been denied and excommunicated from the dominant narrative of the community's educational history could be "spoken."

Psychoanalytic interventions and trauma

Psychoanalysis has a long-standing tradition of intervention with individuals who have experienced trauma. Beginning with *Studies in Hysteria* (1895) Freud postulated that unresolved trauma was at the heart of many patients' current symptoms. The founding paradigm of psychoanalysis is work with patients to reengage trauma, partly by removing the barriers of repression and other defenses that keep trauma disconnected from awareness. Indeed, the idea that engagement with unconscious, repressed traumatic experience is a key to psychological healing remains a central tenet of the theory despite the myriad revisions and transformations that psychoanalysis has undergone since Freud's time (Blum, 2003).

There is a second psychoanalytic narrative of therapeutic intervention that is related to, but which differs from, Freud's Topographical Model, namely, the psychoanalytic understanding that the very process of putting experience into words is therapeutic because language facilitates catharsis and helps organize, objectify, and bind affects that are otherwise overwhelming (Loewenstein, 1956). The expression of thoughts and feelings about meaningful, defining events that have shaped his experience is part of what helps an individual regain his life following emotional devastation. Similarly, Bion (1962) underscored the essential value of putting a powerful experience into words as a means of containing and assimilating the experience, especially when it involves trauma that is otherwise too overwhelming to be digested.

Bohleber (2007) argues that as psychoanalytic interests in the last century, rather than remaining focused on objective trauma, increasingly turned to the inner world of the patient and the here-and-now of the therapeutic relationship via transference and countertransference, catastrophic events, such as the two World Wars and the Holocaust, kept the issues of remembering and remembrance central to the problem of working through, and moving forward from, the aftermath of psychically catastrophic experiences. In fact, some forms of collective trauma, Bohleber argues, turn "remembrance into a special moral requirement" (p. 331). Here memory, recollection, and commemoration are essential to the healing process not because they unearth repressed contents but because they acknowledge lived realities. Curative processes work through acts of testimony. This notion is closely related to collective interventions that focus on the public testimonials of people who have been victims of trauma, such as the truth and reconciliation commissions (TRCs) in South Africa, Guatemala, and elsewhere (see Felman and Laub, 1992). The TRCs are an especially pertinent parallel as they focus on notions of repair, identity, and the reestablishment of a sense of agency following devastating, overwhelming collective experiences (Caruth, 1996; Fullard and Rousseau, 2009). I am arguing here that interventions such as the TRCs, in their multiple functions as cathartic events that also give testimony to unspeakable events, are a form of collective intervention that is related to psychoanalytic ideas about the importance of representation and memory in healing processes.

In reference to the September 11, 2001, attacks on the World Trade Center, Altman and Davies (2002) note that attempting to give shape and meaning to those events is "a daunting and multilayered task" (p. 359), partly because such trauma represents at once a personal and a collective loss. In particular they note that the September 11 attacks created an "emotional/cognitive quagmire" (p. 359), not only for patients who experienced them but also for us as analysts. While clinicians are accustomed to working with childhood trauma and even adult trauma, the shared, collective trauma of 9/11 poses challenges to psychoanalysts in relation to our understanding of what we have to offer those who are most deeply affected by this kind of trauma. The present contribution attempts to illustrate one answer to that question via a description of three interventions.

The community of Hempstead, Texas

Hempstead is fifty miles west of Houston in East Texas, the part of the state that historically and culturally has the strongest affinities with the Old South (as opposed to the rest of Texas, where the influences—and conflicts—have more to do with the state's Spanish and Mexican history). Until the Civil War, cotton plantations and the institution of slavery were the foundations of the area's economy. Present-day Hempstead is almost evenly divided between White and Black residents.[2] A significant part of the town's economy depends on local farming and ranching—town boosters promote it as "the watermelon capital of the world"—and the rest of the residents either own small businesses or commute to jobs in the greater Houston area.

I initially came to Hempstead with an interest in conducting an educational ethnography following a racially charged incident that had pitted the Black community against the Hempstead Independent School District (HISD). I started conducting interviews with educational leaders in the community as well as with parents whose children attended Hempstead High School. In the fall of 1995, during my initial visit, Leory Singleton, who a few years earlier had concluded his tenure as the first Black mayor of the town, pointed out a sign on the side of a building where it was evident that a door had been bricked in, as the more recent brickwork contrasted with the faded bricks of the original structure. Above the bricked-in door, still visible in blocked, white letters, was the word "COLORED." It marked the entrance to which Blacks had once been relegated when entering what was then an eating establishment. More than thirty years after the passage of the Civil Rights Act, this vestige of Jim Crow remained, in plain sight, on the most heavily traveled street of this small town of 3,500 residents.

The Sam Schwarz School

Rural schools in Texas were consolidated in the 1920s. For Black students in the south, this process was facilitated by the Rosenwald Foundation, which hired architects from Tuskegee University to design schools and offered to help underwrite their construction on the condition that local communities donate land as well as matching funds to complete construction. The Rosenwald Schools, as they were known, had a profound impact on Black education in the south during Jim Crow, and the Sam Schwarz School in Hempstead was one of those that benefited from the foundation's vision.

By most accounts, the Sam Schwarz School was successful despite the many challenges its students and their families faced within the community. Nearby Prairie View A&M University had a well-respected school of education that produced excellent teachers, which meant that good teachers staffed the Sam Schwarz School. Many alumni eventually became leaders in Texas and elsewhere. The school also served as a community center, as it was the only venue large enough to host the Black community since Jim Crow laws disallowed the use of other facilities in town. The fact that it played so vital a social and educational role gave the school a special place in the hearts of most of Hempstead's Black residents. The attachment to the school was powerful and evidenced by the fact that almost every time I interviewed a Black parent, she spontaneously referred to the Sam Schwarz School as the cornerstone of the community during Jim Crow.

On method

In the early 1990s I began doing what I have come to term "psychoanalytic ethnography" in communities in Texas and in Mexico (see Ainslie, 1995; 2004; and Ainslie, 2013). These projects were conducted in communities that have been sites of significant conflict and trauma. I used books, films, and photographic exhibits to depict or convey the emotional contours of the situations I encountered in these communities. I view my work as situated within the tradition of psychoanalysis as it existed prior to the great psychoanalytic diaspora that took place in relation to the Second World War. Russell Jacoby (1983) has eloquently described the fact that many analysts at the time were public intellectuals and public in their social activism. Viewed in this light, "activism" includes the process of articulating insights, of putting into words and, sometimes, into representational form (through a variety of media), the understandings that one has drawn from what one has seen, heard, and felt as a psychoanalyst. These insights and understandings are fed and organized by the universe of ideas and sensibilities that defines psychoanalysis. In addition, my approach to interviews draws heavily from the open-ended, free associative stance toward interviews conducted in my consulting room.

Over the course of eighteen months, I spent two to three days in Hempstead every month to six weeks, unless events in the town dictated a different schedule. My aim was to get to know the community. I attended the Waller County Fair, the Hempstead Watermelon Festival, and the Juneteenth Celebrations marking the day when Texas's slaves learned of the Emancipation Proclamation. I attended services in Black churches and I subscribed to *The Waller County News Citizen*, the local newspaper. I also made regular visits to the newspaper's archive.

During my time in Hempstead I conducted many interviews and in the course of this initial work discovered that within Hempstead's Black community there was considerable ambivalence about the current educational climate. This was not surprising; there had been academic research as well as media coverage of this fact. What I had not anticipated, however, was the extent of the lingering feeling about the manner in which the desegregation of schools in Hempstead had been carried out beginning in 1967, when the parents and, in some instances, grandparents of the children currently attending schools within HISD were attending segregated schools in the community. The consistency with which this theme emerged in the preliminary interviews and the emotions often contained in these interviews, led me to focus more specifically on school desegregation and to seek and explore accounts of this experience in interviews.

My interviews repeatedly pointed me in the direction of the Black community's experience of the closing of the Sam Schwarz School, the community's cornerstone since its opening in 1928. Over a period of months, I conducted interviews wherever people felt comfortable: driving around town in their vehicles, in their homes, in city parks, at barbecue establishments, in diners, or at the local Dairy Queen. When it became clear that my research would focus on the experience of school desegregation, I applied to Humanities Texas (the Texas arm of the National Endowment for the Humanities) for a media grant to film a documentary about Hempstead's experience of school desegregation. It should be noted that I received no compensation for any of the work related to this project. That grant underwrote the production costs for *Crossover: A Story of Desegregation* (Ainslie, 1999), a 55-minute film.

While working on the film, I soon discovered that there were many more people who wished to be interviewed than I could possibly use in *Crossover*. The powerful character of many of these interviews led me to try to create a framework within which I could interview a larger number of Sam Schwarz alumni about their experiences during the time of school desegregation. These interviews might be thought of as oral histories, or as forms of *testimonio* (drawing from the Latin American tradition of the personal account of somebody who has been a victim of violence), or as related to the tradition of the TRCs: they were powerful retellings of what it was like to live under the dark shadow of Jim Crow in America's South. After the minister of one of the larger Black churches offered the use of his church as a venue for the interviews, I brought several members of my research team from the University of Texas to Hempstead. They were all doctoral students in Counseling Psychology (the team consisted of one Black, one Latino, and three White students). We spent two weekends conducting interviews with the school's alumni on Saturday and Sunday afternoons.

The therapeutics of *testimonio* and bearing witness

The interviews with Sam Schwarz alumni were emotionally quite powerful. Many of the alumni brought photographs, yearbooks, and other mementos—spontaneous acts that expressed their profound attachment to the school. One man, who had graduated in 1957, pulled his leather-bound diploma from a bag to show me. While several people were waiting to be interviewed, one woman was so moved by the process that she felt compelled to stand and sing the school song. Others in the room cried in response to the gesture. It is difficult to capture fully the experience of listening to these accounts; they were deeply moving and there was an intense desire on the part of many to come to the church to be interviewed, to give testimony in honor of a cherished institution that had played such an important, foundational role in their lives. My team and I were overwhelmed by the wide community participation in these interviews and the outpouring of emotion that we witnessed.

This first intervention in Hempstead was related to the genre of *testimonio* and the methodology of the TRCs as well as to the psychoanalytic commitment to listening to narratives of pain, loss, and conflict. The interviews provided a vessel through which a community's cumulative grievances and mourning found expression. The project had created a space within which narratives of a collective trauma could be told.[3] These narratives included recollections by Black students who lived on the farms and ranches around Hempstead, of having to walk miles to get to school, while neighboring White students were picked up by a school bus, and of helping their principal unload new text books at the train station and then taking them to the White school and bringing discarded, tattered books from the White school back to Sam Schwarz School. The school's football team did not have sufficient equipment to field a full team; the school's basement flooded with every significant rain and the basketball court's floor was dirt. A vignette that was repeated by numerous interviewees told of seeing their esteemed principal working a second job at night, mopping floors at a car dealership. Following desegregation, one student remembered taking a drink from the water fountain at school and then seeing a White student wipe it off before drinking from it.

The narratives that emerged from these interviews captured experiences of collective devaluation. They were infused with anger at the injustices suffered and mourning at the loss of a cherished, transference-laden institution; the Sam Schwarz School had "held" the Black community in a variety of vital, important ways. The school had fostered a broad sense of community, which many believed was now lost. Part of what surprised me in the narratives was the profound sense of loss that many felt, the sense that the Black community had paid an unacknowledged cost during the Civil Rights era. To a degree that most of the rest of the country could not appreciate, much less understand, there was a sense that social progress had come at the Black community's expense. This first intervention, then, was in the creation of a forum for these experiences to be voiced and shared.

The *Crossover* film drew from a subset of the church interviews as well as from other interviews (the individuals who were interviewed at the church, and whose accounts became part of the film, were subsequently reinterviewed while the church interviews were only audiotaped). However, unlike the church interviews, the film became a public document or representation, and thus I consider it a second, albeit related, intervention. *Crossover* was screened in many Texas communities, as well as at conferences and public events in other parts of the country. It was through the film that the *testimonio* or TRC elements of these stories became a public, shared experience. (Despite repeated efforts I was unsuccessful in my efforts to screen the film in Hempstead. However, many Blacks traveled to Houston and to Austin to attend screenings.)

Reengaging exiled narratives

Beyond the "Colored" sign above the bricked-in door that in 1995 could still be read by anyone who happened to look, there remained countless examples of conscious and unconscious racism in Hempstead. They constituted macro- and microaggressions (Sue et al., 2007) that formed part of the fabric of daily life.

Every trace of the Sam Schwarz School had been erased. Without consultation, the building itself was razed after Hempstead's schools were desegregated, despite the fact that it was an important landmark for the Black community. As described in *Crossover*, most of the contents of the school, including a trove of trophies that personified generations of Jim Crow era successes in scholastic and athletic competition, simply vanished. (Some in the community claimed that the trophies had been summarily loaded up and taken to the city dump. Others claimed that the memorabilia had been stored by school officials, only to be destroyed by vandals. The only consensus was that the trophies had indeed disappeared.) For many Blacks, the fate of the trophies became emblematic of their experience and confirmed that Whites had no regard or respect for anything that the Black community valued.

The official HISD history contained no account of the Sam Schwarz School or of its closing.

During present-day HISD sporting events, when Jim Crow era classes were honored ("We want to recognize Hempstead High School's class of 1960") there was no mention of the Sam Schwarz School alumni.

Hempstead High School continued the practice, begun at the time of school desegregation, of electing separate White and Black homecoming queens.

At the site where the Sam Schwarz School had stood there was nothing to mark it as a place of historical significance. The school district initially built a new junior high school at the location and that campus was renamed. A new junior high school was later built elsewhere, at which point the HISD decided to house students who had academic and behavior problems at the original Sam Schwarz site. Incredibly, in an act of unconscious or deliberate racism, *this* school was named the Sam Schwarz Campus. It was the first time since the school's closing that the name had been used. In other words, the school district had chosen to use the cherished name for the campus where it was housing its problem students. Understandably, the Black community was incensed.

Chosen traumas and chosen glories

Vamik Volkan (1997) has used the terms "chosen trauma" and "chosen glory" to capture what he views as two essential elements of collective experience that contribute to group identity. (By "chosen" Volkan makes clear that he does not mean that they are literally selected, but rather that they are invoked in conscious and unconscious ways as part of collective identity processes.) Chosen traumas are collective, shared mental representations of traumatic events that have befallen a group and which remain unresolved or incompletely mourned. Often, they are handed down to subsequent generations in conscious and unconscious ways as psychological tasks to be resolved or as emotional wounds to be repaired. Chosen traumas are complex psychological processes that are activated and played out in a variety of ways, but it is their linkage to individual and group identity that makes chosen traumas especially potent as collective psychic organizers.

Similarly, chosen glories are shared mental representations of collective experiences that capture a group's sense of pride. For this reason they, too, are important elements in shaping collective identity. Members of a group participate in the feelings of triumph or accomplishment that are captured in the chosen glory.

Both of these constructs were helpful to me in conceptualizing what I gradually came to learn about the demise of the Sam Schwarz School, as well as the meaning of the school for Hempstead's Black residents. It was apparent that the school represented both a chosen trauma and a chosen glory for Hempstead's Black community. This dual status was reflected in the fact that in interview after interview the school was repeatedly invoked, both as a painful loss and as a point of deep pride. It also represented a narcissistic wound: the one institution (excluding Hempstead's Black churches) that embodied the Black community's aspirations had been treated as just so much rubble following the demise of Jim Crow. The disappearance of the school's trophies was symbolic of an experience of collective devaluation. The feelings of loss were clearly not about a wish to return to Jim Crow, they were about losing a vital institution that had helped the community endure the ravages of devaluation and dehumanization.

At the time of desegregation few in the Black community could fathom the ways in which social progress would come at their expense—that the hard-fought attainments of the Civil Rights era would mean, for example, that countless Black teachers and coaches would lose their jobs. (Although a few Black teachers were allowed to "cross over," many White parents were resistant to the idea of Blacks teaching their children, and Whites controlled the school boards.) The Sam Schwarz School was not integrated into the system; it was closed and its legacy erased (one alumnus summed it up noting that not only had the school been razed, but its colors, mascot, and song had also all been left behind). The final insult was that, after Jim Crow, tracking resulted in the resegregation of Black students, now within the same school building.

On the other hand, there appeared to be denial and/or indifference within Hempstead's White community regarding the cost that the Black community had incurred during school desegregation. For some, there was even a detectable resentment, as if Blacks had been "given" so much and yet were still not satisfied. Most younger Whites had little or no understanding of this history within their own community; indeed, many, if not most, had never heard of the Sam Schwarz School, every trace of which had disappeared more than a decade before they were born. As was evident from the Black interviews, however, the Black community had not forgotten.

The Sam Schwarz School represented both a chosen trauma and a chosen glory in Volkan's sense. It was a chosen glory in that the institution had been a bulwark against the aggressions and humiliations of Jim Crow, an enclave within which Black educators were valued and respected and where the community could gather. It was a chosen trauma because the school's demise, and the obvious devaluation that permitted White authorities to erase every trace of the school from the community's official memory, left a deep, festering wound within the Black community.

The third intervention

My work in Hempstead had been organized around two aims: the gathering of *testimonios* or oral histories of the alumni and the creation of a documentary film to depict this experience. The third aim was to develop a community intervention aimed at speaking to the underlying tensions and disavowed history within the community. Using another grant from Humanities Texas, I organized a public program in Hempstead that would name what had remained unnamed, that would attempt to reengage what was disavowed, and that would perhaps help attenuate the underlying anger that comes when powerful experiences of humiliation and loss go unacknowledged. I conceived of this third intervention as a kind of psychoanalytic interpretation: the articulation of underlying conflicts with the aim of helping engage and connect experiences, partly by bringing aspects of the past into a clearer focus and awareness and partly by using the power of language and representation to help heal wounds. In other words, there was a twofold strategy at work. In relation to Hempstead's Black community, the aim was to foster a process whereby there could be a public, collective acknowledgement of the chosen trauma/chosen glory character of the experiences surrounding the Sam Schwarz School. That included affirming the value of what the White community had mostly seen in devalued terms. Second, the intervention was also a vehicle for voicing the bitter truths of the school desegregation process, a historical moment that Whites tended to view narrowly, and sometimes grudgingly, as a time when the proponents of Civil Rights had had their way, without seeing the cost to the Black community of that success and, more concretely, the emotional complexity of this experience from a Black perspective. In this effort, I was keenly aware that the *framing* of the "interpretation" would mean everything in terms of whether or not it could be heard or "used."

Enlisting the participation of key Sam Schwarz alumni, I formed a committee that would play a vital role in fashioning the intervention. This committee (a dozen people in all, including, among others: the minister of one of the most important Black churches; a revered Black educator who had attended Sam Schwarz as a child, had taught there during desegregation, and who had subsequently become the first Black teacher at Hempstead

High School; a well-known White teacher who had taught in the district during desegregation; a Black school board member; and the White superintendent of HISD) helped shape the intervention in ways that would be meaningful to both the Black and the White community.

The intervention was called "The Sam Schwarz Reunion and Retrospective." It was held on September 26, 1998, a Saturday morning, at an HISD facility. Black participation was mobilized through Black churches, informal alumni networks, and word of mouth. Several strategies were devised to encourage the attendance of Hempstead's White community: the school district's teachers were given in-service training credit for attending the program, middle-school and high-school art classes designed the sets and students' art projects related to Hempstead's history were on display. The elementary school and high school choirs also performed. The hope was that, if for no other reason, White parents would come to see their children's artwork and performances. These strategies were successful: the audience was racially mixed, with significant White attendance.

There were several highlights of the event, which was given ample coverage in *The Waller County News Citizen.* The school district issued a proclamation marking the day Sam Schwarz School Day. Sam Schwarz teachers, administrators, and alumni were recognized and the choirs sang the school's song. In an especially meaningful gesture, the school district set up two permanent display cases in its offices at the site of the original school. (The in-school suspension program had by now been moved elsewhere and the school district had moved its offices to the site, which retained the name "Sam Schwarz Campus.") Alumni had donated photographs and memorabilia that were to be on permanent display. My task was to describe the era of school desegregation as a collective trauma drawing from the dozens of interviews my students and I had done regarding the demise of the Sam Schwarz School. A leading Black scholar at the University of Texas gave a gripping presentation on "Contemporary Issues in Education," in which he addressed race as a vital challenge for educators. Finally, several distinguished alumni spoke: James Anderson, Ph.D., Dean of the College of Engineering at North Carolina State University; General Kemp Hilliard, M.D., a cardiac surgeon in San Francisco; and Paul Menifee, M.D., the first Black pediatric surgeon in the state of Texas. Their talks were powerful and moving and certified the idea that despite the collective humiliations of Jim Crow and the pervasive shortage of resources (virtually everything at the school, from books to laboratory equipment, to athletic equipment, was a hand-me-down from the district's White schools), many of the school's alumni had gone on to make significant contributions to society. In other words, the structure of the program was such that the teachers and alumni celebrated the school as a chosen glory, whereas it fell to me to speak to the school's demise as a chosen trauma. That was by design, and the committee was unanimous in the view that, as an outsider and as a faculty member of a respected university, I was the appropriate person to speak of the things that I had learned in my interviews regarding the experience of school desegregation in their community.

The afternoon was reserved for Sam Schwarz School class reunions and the first school-wide reunion since the school was razed in the late 1960s.

Concluding considerations

The documentary film and the process of collecting *testimonios* drew heavily from psychoanalytic notions about the therapeutic value of putting words to experience, of speaking that which is otherwise too painful to speak. The third intervention drew from psychoanalytic ideas about the importance of making conscious that which is unconscious and/or excommunicated and disavowed; bringing it into engagement with the present.

The intervention in Hempstead was intended to address a chosen trauma and a chosen glory that played an important role in the Black community's self-understanding and in White–Black relations within the community at large. The fate of the school was itself symbolic of a broader range of experiences to which the Black community was subjected during Jim Crow and subsequent to the passage of the Civil Rights Act. Neither I nor the Hempstead group that comprised the organizing committee for the Sam Schwarz Reunion and Retrospective had any illusions that this intervention could undo the many complex and deep-seated emotions that lingered in this community and that linked acts of violence, racism, and humiliation to identity processes and inter-group tensions in profound ways. As with any interpretation, the aim was more modest: to foster reflection and acknowledgement in hopes that through such processes the emotional geographies of the White and Black communities might find openings for more constructive engagement. This intervention created discussion within the community—that much is certain. In addition, there were tangible results: a plaque commemorating the Sam Schwarz School was placed at the site of the old school, in the school district's offices, along with the two trophy cases that contained memorabilia describing the school and the lives it held. Alumni of the school had their first reunion since the school's demise (perhaps a symptom of the fragmentation that accompanies traumatic experiences). And, lastly, someone took a ladder down to Hempstead's main street and painted over the "Colored" sign above the bricked-in entrance that had once been the only way in which Blacks could get service at the establishment. Admittedly, these accomplishments were probably modest in scope and impact. But I would argue that they nevertheless contributed to a meaningful and constructive engagement with events that continued to haunt the community in the present. Like every meaningful interpretation, the intervention fostered engagement with important issues. It is the absence of such engagement that fuels polarization and festering social conflict.

Notes

1 Reprinted from *Psychoanalysis, Culture & Society, suppl. Special Issue: Psychoanalysis, Trauma, and Community* 18.2 (Jun 2013): 140–152 by permission of Palgrave Macmillan.
2 Following the American Psychological Association guidelines for avoiding racial/ethnic bias in language, I have adopted the convention of capitalizing "Black" and "White" to designate individuals of African-American and European-American ancestry, respectively.
3 I am indebted to Elizabeth Goren and Judith Alpert for helping me understand my work through this lens.

References

Ainslie, R.C. (1995) *No Dancin' in Anson: An American Story of Race and Social Change*. New York: Jason Aronson, Inc.

Ainslie, R.C. (Dir.) (1999) *Crossover: A Story of Desegregation* [documentary film]. Austin: Dos Manos Productions.

Ainslie, R.C. (2004) *Long Dark Road: The Story of Bill King and Jasper's Murder*. Austin: University of Texas Press.

Ainslie, R.C. (2013) *The Fight to Save Juárez: Life in the Heart of Mexico's Drug War*. Austin: University of Texas Press.

Altman, N. and Davies, J. (2002) Out of the blue: Reflections on a shared trauma. *Psychoanalytic Dialogues* 12(3): 359–360.

Bion, W.R. (1962) A psycho-analytic study of thinking. *International Journal of Psychoanalysis* 43: 306–310.

Blum, H. (2003) Psychic trauma and traumatic object loss. *Journal of the American Psychoanalytic Association* 51(2): 415–432.

Bohleber, W. (2007) Remembrance, trauma and collective memory: The battle for memory in psychoanalysis. *International Journal of Psychoanalysis* 88 (2): 329–352.

Breuer, J. and Freud, S. (1893–1895). *Studies on Hysteria*. In *The Standard Edition of the Complete Psychological Works of Sigmund Freud*, Vol. II. Translated and edited by J. Strachey. London: Hogarth Press, 1955.

Caruth, C. (1996) *Unclaimed Experience: Trauma, Narrative, and History*. Baltimore: Johns Hopkins University Press.

Felman, S. and Laub, D. (1992) *Testimony: Crises of Witnessing in Literature, Psychoanalysis, History*. New York: Routledge.

Fullard, M. and Rousseau, N. (2009) *Truth-Telling, Identities and Power in South Africa and Guatemala*. New York: International Center for Transitional Justice.

Jacoby, R. (1983) *The Repression of Psychoanalysis*. Chicago and London: University of Chicago Press.

Loewenstein, R.M. (1956) Some remarks on the role of speech in psychoanalytic technique. *International Journal of Psycho-Analysis* 37 (3): 460–468.

Sue, D.W., Capodilupo, C.M., Torino, C., Bucceri, J.M., Holder, A.M.B., Nadal, K.L. and Esquilin, M. (2007) Racial microaggressions in everyday life: Implications for clinical practice. *American Psychologist* 62 (4): 271–286.

Volkan, V.D. (1997) *Blood Lines: From Ethnic Pride to Ethnic Terrorism*. Boulder: Westview Press.

Chapter 7

Beyond "thank you for your service"

The creation of post-war veteran/non-veteran collaborative mourning spaces

Donna Bassin

A note on inspiration

This chapter is an expansion of an essay I wrote for a portfolio of fine art prints and essays in 2014, *Celebrate People's History: Iraq Veterans Against the War*, a collaboration between some 60 veteran and non-veteran artists and writers to commemorate Iraq Veterans Against the War's (IVAW) ten-year anniversary. Collaboration is the thread of the current chapter: in theme, subject material, its very composition, and its nascent end goal. Many of the following words have been given to me by the veterans who have been generous enough to let me follow their journey—words heard in many conversations and interviews from participants of Combat Paper New Jersey workshops, or found in the poetry of Warrior Writers,[1] two of the most active organizations in the emerging veterans' art movement.[2] I have also asked Kevin Basl, an Iraq War veteran and facilitator with both organizations, to carefully read what I have written, in order to maintain respect for the cultures of the military and veterans in the telling of their stories. To get close to these veterans is to be touched and inspired. They have let me into their community to film them, interview them, listen to their stories, and make art with them and for that I am grateful.

Over the past decade, my work and the numerous relations I've made with veterans have pulled me further away from the traditional clinical setting and deeper into community work. This chapter (perhaps too ambitiously) is my attempt to work through aspects of veterans' struggles to "come back home," share some of their restorative efforts in this journey, and contribute to a growing practice of psychoanalytically minded community mental health workers, while also reflecting on my own professional changes following 9/11. The conclusion I've drawn through my decade-plus field study is currently a work in progress: a warehouse-sized art installation—a collaborative mourning space—entitled By Our Own Hand, set to be opened in 2016. Beyond offering a detailed description of that project, this chapter will provide a summary of the path—the relationships, the materials, the lessons learned—leading to the development of such a space.

Overcoming resistance to the "violence of silence": Post Traumatic Stress and moral injury

Initially, I was a curious bystander to a number of veterans' movements, post-9/11. I observed as they transformed themselves from bystanders to witnesses of their own war-torn selves. I also observed different restorative and redemptive mourning practices in a number of the veteran communities, all of which had committed themselves to social activism, advocacy for wounded warriors at home, sponsorship of memorializing rituals for those killed in action or "missing in action," and self-witnessing through the creation of art and poetry. Over time, the therapeutic wisdom of the veterans' art and social justice movements became apparent, not only for their own journeys but for my own professional goals and personal development. I wanted to learn from their experiences and bring their insights and practices to the public.

My original interest was in the deconstruction of the "coming home" or "coming back to self and civilian relationships" practices of veterans' communities hoping to enrich our contemporary psychoanalytic understanding of catastrophic grief and (the working-through processes of) mourning, as well as resilience and self-forgiveness. More recently my attention has shifted to working collaboratively with Combat Paper NJ in their endeavor to create conditions for self-witnessing and subsequently share veterans' stories with the majority of the non-veteran civilian population who has no visceral experiences with the damages and violence of war. Of course, we all condemn war and the monstrosity of the crimes we commit against each other; however, for the most part, the American public unfortunately remains a bystander to the violence of war, and the violence our veterans hold both as victims and as perpetrators. As bystanders, it is possible to commit a "violence of silence," perpetrated by remaining inattentive to our shared responsibility for violence committed in our name by our warrior class. We non-veteran civilians need their stories and images of war to be able to begin the necessary task of witness, a civic responsibility as well as a social–psychological. Hannah Segel (1997) asserts that psychoanalysts who believe in the therapeutic power of speech must not be silent in the face of human suffering. This cessation of the violence of silence is a shared mission.

For many of the veterans I've met and worked with over the past decade, mourning has not been a private affair; they have taken on acts of social responsibility and humanitarian action, publicly sharing their inner battles and those memories that haunt them. Their exposure to the best and worst aspects of human experience—love and aggression—and their telling has triggered my own sense of vulnerability and, as Butler (2004, 2014) has speculated, slowly transformed me into a witness that is compelled to take action.

Over the past decade of war, the therapeutic wisdom of the veterans' art and social justice movements have become clearer in my mind. Their work requires an ongoing practice to learn how to take in and then "stay with," rather than turn away from, their testimonies of war. While many of them struggle to witness the catastrophic impact of war, they continue to carry a burden, an inner war that will remain with many of them for the rest of their lives. Like a Greek chorus, the stories our veterans carry express our collective sorrow; bearing culpability and trauma, they warn of the dangers of ignoring and forgetting. They hold the grief of war for us who will not. But they also hold something the majority of the US population remains unaware of: the bonds of loving attachments, connection (and camaraderie) constructed in the face of collective exposure to violence, death, and when the fog lifts, survivorship. For the ancient Greeks, it is these relational bonds that served as a ground when they and those around them went mad during combat (Shay, 1994, 1995, 2002).

Upon coming home from war, many veterans and service members find themselves in battle with a new enemy, Post Traumatic Stress (PTS). While existing protocols for the treatment of PTS have been useful for many returning veterans, others have received little help, being given a handful of prescriptions and barely a counseling session. Please note, that I have chosen to use Post Traumatic Stress rather than Post Traumatic Stress Disorder in order to de-pathologize what in fact is a human response to war rather than an adjustment disorder. Some of the veterans I have worked with speak of PTS as a portal only to gain access to whatever health benefits the US Department of Veterans Affairs offers. And still others perceive the diagnostic category as a negation of the complexity of their experiences and a disavowal of the collective responsibility of the entire citizen population (veterans and non-veterans alike) to bear the burden of the sequelae of war. They are resistant to the idea that reactions to the horrors of war should be seen as an adjustment disorder when in fact, as veteran Jeremy Stainthorp Berggren, a former Marine in mortuary affairs and active performer with Warrior Writers, states in simple terms in his poem, "P.lease T.ry S.omething D.ifferent," "try seeing death and then have nothing go wrong" (2011). Suicide, alcoholism, drug addiction, and isolation are solutions for many combat veterans who have killed or watched horrific violence.

The US Department of Veterans Affairs now recognizes moral injury as an additional aspect of the stresses of war, often accompanying PTS. Jonathan Shay (1994, 1995, 2002) has extensively studied the narratives and traumas of the Vietnam veteran, and in his close readings of *The Iliad* and *The Odyssey*, first observed moral injury in veterans, and began to refer to it as "something more than PTSD." Litz et al. (2009) have extended Shay's observations with research concerning the grave psychological ramifications for military personnel perpetrating or witnessing acts that violate collectively shared moral beliefs. They have concluded that the sequelae of moral injury and ethical conflicts can't be understood within our current conceptualization of Post Traumatic Stress Disorder.

From my couch to the streets—"The Ride to Freedom" and "Walkin' to New Orleans"

Following 9/11, as a consultant to the mayor's office of New York City, I was "assigned" to develop bereavement strategies for the grieving families of the victims and help facilitate the mourning process of a terrorized and grieving city. My experience at the devastated site where the World Trade Towers had stood, inside Ground Zero, was visceral. Being inside this violated and dismembered space evoked terror, anguish, and grief. I felt under siege trying to think in what could only be called a war zone. I spent too much time in the devastation of Ground Zero and left emotionally wounded and professionally challenged. Looking for support from others who had seen the ruins of war and seeking new models of community mourning after collective catastrophic loss, I left the protected sanctity of the consulting room, and soon after I turned to combat veterans of the wars in Vietnam, Afghanistan, and Iraq for their wisdom in coping with such profound trauma. I eventually found my way to extended nighttime conversations with veterans, many of them members of Rolling Thunder, Inc., who were confronting their pasts at the Vietnam Veterans Memorial Wall in Washington, D.C. My initial visits were viewed with a certain suspicion and resistance to speaking with me. But over a three-year period of showing up at their events and listening to political views and concerns they slowly accepted my presence.

While supporting the US commitment to the wars in Iraq and Afghanistan, Rolling Thunder, Inc., consisting mainly of veterans who served in Vietnam, demonstrate against the US government's ongoing negligence of our returning warriors. A large part of their manifest agenda is the protest against the US government's lack of effort in seeking those "prisoners of war" and "missing in action" from the Vietnam War. They have also been insistent in getting government support for the recovery of "old bones" hoping to provide closure and permission to grieve to families who have never been absolutely certain of the death of their loved ones or able to bury remains. Annually, over Memorial Day weekend in Washington, D.C, as many as half a million Harley-Davidson motorcycles ride in remembrance and in protest from the North Parking lot of the Pentagon around the city to Maya Lin's Vietnam Veterans Memorial Wall. The pipes of these motorcycles create their own rolling thunder, echoing the sounds of helicopters and B-52 bombers, perhaps reminiscent of the organization's namesake 1965 bombing campaign against North Vietnam, "Operation Rolling Thunder." This parade, the "Ride for Freedom," has transformed Memorial Day for these veterans, reclaiming it from the traditional, however limited, military displays of honor and from the barbecues and picnics that celebrate the start of summer. In essence, The Ride disavows the losses associated with the creation of this once meaningful remembrance day. In the process of constructing their own welcome home parade they have attempted to bring veterans down to the Wall to help them confront unresolved pasts and to initiate a healing process. Over the years, more and more Vietnam veterans have made the pilgrimage to the Wall. Veterans refer to those who come to see the Wall but stay at the edge of trees surrounding it as "50 yarders" or "tree liners," those yet to allow themselves to walk into the memorial's center where anguished memories might be evoked.[3] More or less aware of their own war-torn, dissociate selves, many remain metaphorically "prisoners of war" and still "missing in action." Collectively attempting to affect their own return they have sought to communalize traumatic loss through strong relational ties with other veterans, creating their own facilitating environments in which to access complicated losses and manage the grief of war. Artie Muller, a Vietnam veteran and head of the New Jersey Chapter of Rolling Thunder, Inc. has described these deep platonic bonds among soldiers, observing that often even gravely injured soldiers want to return to war, because their brothers and sisters are "there." He has said you fight together, you die together, you share whatever you have and furthermore if you haven't been in that situation you just won't understand" (Bassin, 2008, 2014). Shay (1994, 1995) has also emphasized the deep passion among those who experience combat together, comparing it to the earliest, profound family attachments. Society's failure to acknowledge this intimacy and love between soldiers during war, amplifies the veterans' isolation and solitude. Veterans come back to the civilian world where they are no longer held in the strong relational field they served within.

After a number of Memorial Day weekends with Rolling Thunder, Inc., I would meet Jan Barry, grassroots activist, poet, and journalist. In his quiet wisdom, he pointed me toward the work of a manifestly different group of veterans: Veterans for Peace (VFP), IVAW, and Vietnam Veterans Against the War (VVAW), an organization Barry co-founded in 1967. Barry was instrumental in eliciting Robert Lifton's participation in the original veterans' self-help groups and served as my mentor and introduced me to many of those at the helm of the veterans groups.

On the third anniversary of the post-9/11 US invasion of Iraq, I had the honor to join, as a civilian participant and documentarian, a five-day, 132-mile trek along the Gulf Coast, on Highway 90 from Mobile, Alabama, to New Orleans: "The Veterans' and Survivors' March." This simultaneous act of witness, protest, pilgrimage, and reparation was conceived by the older generation of veterans from VVAW and VFP who, as David Cline (then National President of VFP) suggested, had re-emerged with new force to protest the war in Iraq and provide guidance to returning Iraq vets who founded IVAW in 2004. David told me that he, like many Vietnam-era veterans, felt disbelief and enormous frustration over the nation's abandonment of its returning military personnel after war's end, and took this repetition "as a slap in the face." With a legitimacy and authority only possible by their own military service and recollections of the young soldiers they once were, the Vietnam-era vets stood in as concerned and compassionate parents to the newly returned Iraq War veterans. For many Vietnam-era veterans, the temporal boundary between the wars on terror and Vietnam had dissolved. Increased numbers of the older veterans came out of their isolation and began to acknowledge ongoing and long-term struggles with a variety of post-combat stress and losses. The War on Terror triggered, as Toni Morrison (1987) suggests in her novel *Beloved*, disremembered pasts that are haunted by that which was neither forgotten nor remembered. The Vietnam-era veterans also served as interlocutors, providing the initial language and "therapeutic endeavors" for the younger generation. However, like all generative parents, the Vietnam-era veterans gracefully moved over and took a place on the sidelines, empowering IVAW to take leadership.

A moving peace train, with IVAW up front, consisting of VFP, Military Families Speak Out, Gold Star Families for Peace, and Survivors of Hurricane Katrina, walked, danced, gave testimony, and sang reconstructed military cadence to bring national awareness to the traumatic plight of the survivors of Hurricane Katrina and the negligence of the government to care for them. During the march, I heard a number of the younger veterans describe the strong resemblance of the storm-ravaged coast with the devastation they had seen in Iraq. I imagined that, like a homeopathic remedy, a dose of devastated American landscape reignited those losses experienced in combat and resonated with the internal devastation one must feel post-war. But here in the supportive environment of their band of brothers and sisters, grief and vulnerability became rebelliousness, harnessed for social justice. Grief, as I have learned from my contact with many in IVAW, is complicated and often laced with guilt and shame, as many veterans experience themselves not as victims but as perpetrators. And grief, for IVAW, was not marked under marble memorials, but rather used to ignite attempts at restoration and reparation. During the march, Garret Reppenhagen, who had served as a sniper in Iraq before joining IVAW, shared his experience of moral injury. His response is worth quoting at length:

> After I shot my first innocent civilian, I was very distraught. I came back to my bunk, my hooch, and I destroyed it. I tore everything down. I was a mess. There's another form of mental illness that isn't being addressed, and that's the fact that a lot of us are coming back

> and we don't feel like the victim. A lot of us feel like the criminal. We feel like we're the murderer, the thief, we're the rapist, and we come back and it's, "Thank you, Johnny. You did a great job, Johnny. Well done, Johnny. Welcome home, Johnny. Here's a beer, Johnny. Drink one on us, Johnny."
>
> *Leave No Soldier* (Bassin, 2008, 2014)

> And Johnny's somewhere in the Midwest where it's not socially acceptable to say, "Hey, hold the hell on. You guys got it wrong. What I did is not good. I was killing farmers and craftsmen and Iraqis that were upset of the abuse and the humiliation of the occupation." And I'm not getting sent to prison. Now I'm being thanked. I'm guilty for what I did, and the shame is that I'm guilty of who I've become. And if I'm not punished for what I did, then I'm going to punish myself. Whether I'm conscious of it or not. I'm going to get into alcohol and drugs … I'm going to abuse my family and take it out on them, or my friends. I'm going to isolate myself and confine myself. I'm going to hang myself or shoot myself, because I am guilty.

Garret continued to speak of the value of IVAW:

> But with Iraq Veterans Against the War I can take that power back. I empower myself. And that is a huge healing step because there are a lot of soldiers out there that feel like they can't do anything. And they sit in their homes and they rot because they don't realize that there are organizations out there like us. They don't realize that they're not alone and there are other people that feel the same way that they do, and are doing something about it. And that's why I'm here. That's why I'm at the march. That's why I'm frustrated about what happened when the hurricane hit New Orleans and the government did nothing, because I see it happen over and over again to the veterans all the time. There's a lack of responsibility to our citizens. I have to be engaged; I have to try to do well. I've got my third eye opened up and I can't close it now because I've seen the wrong. And if I rest and I stop doing this kind of work, then the war creeps up on me even more. My nightmares get worse.

Here, rage has covered grief and Garret draws a link between self-destructive behaviors and the smothering of pain of grief and self-loathing.

Anne Carson (2006) reminds us, "Why does tragedy exist? Because you are full of rage. Why are you full of rage? Because you are full of grief." Grief, in the context of IVAW, may be seen as rebellious and useful to activate and direct social activism. Service people are taught that at times they must kill or be killed, though as veteran–poet and IVAW member Jon Turner (2014) bluntly reminds us in his poem "Standard Operating Procedure": "No one in their right mind would kill a man." Stan Goff, a former Special Forces sergeant and current anti-war activist, has said military service people in Vietnam were taught to say, "It don't mean anything. We just killed a woman, it don't mean anything. One of our soldiers just got killed, it don't mean anything" (Bassin, 2008, 2014). Boundaries between "them and us," friend and enemy, the living and the dead, must be firm and absolute in the theater of war. But as Goff has also observed, once you put on the psychological armor of detachment, you can't take it off. And in the midst of the fog of war,[4] soldiers find themselves detached from the horrors and may have little or only a vague memory of what happened and what they saw.

The grief of the veterans on the Gulf Coast March unsettled me. But, as Garret suggests, access to such grief can be redemptive and used to build an effective ethical community. For many returning combat soldiers, the grieving self is experienced—despite the overwhelming pain and anguish—as a necessary part of the change that loss and violent actions engender, an embodiment of one's fidelity to remembrance, and a place where attachments to their losses may survive. Clinical interventions that attempt to provide pre-mature narrative suggesting the protective strategy of "moving on" may be experienced as mis-attunement with the complicated and multi-layered experiences, particular of combat veterans who experience themselves, with guilt and shame, as both victims and perpetrators. Many combat veterans are resistant to the misguided but culturally sanctioned idea of "moving on" and "getting over it" and feel banished from the very communities that sent them to war and to whom they must return as sanitized civilians.

While soldiers are battle-proofed and "taught how to kill" as psychological protection, the protective armor (as Goff has described) must come off in order to integrate back to civilian life. But the morally reprehensible acts don't peel off as does the uniform or get left behind on the battlefield, and the grey areas that fall beneath the cracks of the rules of engagement are enormous when combat occurs within a village or city, where civilians and enemy combatants are often interspersed and ambiguity precedes life or death decision-making. "Perpetrating, failing to prevent, or bearing witness to acts that transgress deeply held moral beliefs and expectations" (Litz et al., 2009, p. 697) create within service personnel severe inner conflicts, isolation, shame, guilt, and deep grief for the moral person they were before war. Losses caused by moral injury cut deep into the psyche and may create ongoing inner conflicts.

Many veterans experience confusion about how to mourn this person they now experience themselves no longer to be. While loss is unique and individual, understanding of the loss often requires social validation of the moral transgressions and injuries to the sense of self-worth as well as an empathic non-judgmental community to help the veteran manage the overwhelming affects. How can traumas of moral injury be mitigated through listening—by tolerating the horror of the veterans' stories—not turning away or being apathetic? These veterans call for the creation of a space in which the individual's life as forever changed by the experience of loss and moral injury can be held as an ongoing process. As one changes, the meaning of one's actions hopefully undergoes some compassionate revision initiating the beginning of a long journey toward forgiveness. By perceiving veterans as others placed in a position of either heroes/victims or perpetrators, they have been denied the necessary spaces where losses might be named and mourned.

Most soldiers hold on to an ideal that state-sanctioned violence is a noble cause, to protect their character from the potentially damaging effects. However, over time, that protective bubble will pop. If it is years down the road, the buildup of stress will be more harmful. Whether conscious of it or not, because these soldiers are never punished by society and their leaders are not being held accountable, the veteran takes on self-destructive habits and sometimes commits suicide, as described by Reppenhagen above.

Among the veterans I have worked with there is an attempt to find ethical narratives that transcend the old polarities of victims and perpetuators, as well as a new language that recasts the impact of war on soldiers' hearts and minds from a medical formulation of wounds and disorders. Many vets are left wondering what an appropriate response to the horrific acts of war might be.

Leave no soldier and the bonds of love

Tim O'Brien, Vietnam veteran and author of *The Things They Carried* (1990), has described the heavy loads that combat soldiers carry on the battlefield: weapons, mine detectors, tents, radios, bibles, fear, grief, and most poignantly, each other. This military ethos of "leave no fallen soldier behind" reminds those who serve to honor their humanity, even in the surrealistic theaters of war. Rolling Thunder, Inc., IVAW and its parental communities, VFP and VVAW, have taken this ethos from the battlefield, extended its literal meaning, and applied it to their post-war civilian lives.

The refusal to abandon those still missing in action or to turn away from those lost who symbolically reside on the Vietnam Wall may be seen as an understandable, although melancholia, response to loss. However, the activities of Rolling Thunder, Inc. and Gold Star Mothers (mothers who have lost their children in war) lobbying for changes in veterans' legislation and visiting at US Department of Veterans Affairs hospitals suggests the ability to develop caring relationships in the present simultaneously with a fidelity to the past. Eng and Kazanjian (2003) argue that the refusal to abandon the dead through conventional mourning may be seen as an ethical commitment to love and may demonstrate the useful and rebellious aspects of melancholia. Many of the above veterans' activities suggest that one can both maintain a relationship with their lost loved ones as well as invest in social justice projects and new relationships.

Over the years of my education within these various veterans' communities I came to appreciate the new narratives that were unfolding. These veterans refused to be victims looking for revenge and retaliation and eschewed the unreflective manic response of civilians who wore yellow ribbons and "thanked them for their service." Instead, they have been working to become activists, caregivers, protestors, and restorers. These truly heroic efforts are forms of reparation and self-forgiveness.

As I listened to the stories of the veterans, my awareness of their need for public platforms grew. Edie McCoy, a member of Rolling Thunder, Inc. who was an intensive care nurse in Vietnam, says, "Some people say that the sound of bikes sound like helicopters. I don't think so. I think they sound like power. When you are on these bikes and with the powerful people who drive them, you feel like you finally have some power [to get the nation's attention]" (Bassin, 2008, 2014). I heard many stories similar to McCoy's that spoke to the veterans' efforts to mobilize grief of war and moral injury into humanitarian and moral repair and to have public platforms on which to tell their stories. My interest in creating a public platform on which the wisdom of the veterans could be shared and recognition and compassion inspired, pushed me into creative engagement with the concerns, tasks, and ethics of public witnessing and the power of aesthetic representation. As a psychoanalytic practitioner, attention to the aesthetics of affect regulation and construction of a coherent narrative was well within my experience. As a filmmaker, I was challenged to evoke and represent the testimonies of the veterans in a form that would engage and "move" the audience from bystander to witness without contributing to further injury and suffering or diminishing those whose stories are told. The finished product, *Leave No Soldier* (Bassin, 2008, 2014), bears witness to their efforts, but moreover presents, in coherent story form, alternative narratives of post-war collective grieving.

The ways in which veterans have attempted to carry each other in the service of "leave no soldier behind," to build a community that extends the bonds of attachment and love, the ability to stay in these spaces where past, present, and future exist simultaneously and past loss is metabolized serving as a fertile ground for change, shaped the direction my documentary took. In *Leave No Soldier*, combat veterans and military nurses open their lives to unexpected and potentially transformative possibilities through their commitment to take the military oath—"leave no soldier behind" —from the battlefield to the home front. For many, massive traumatic losses (and those they may have caused) catalyzed a call to activism and social responsibility. Their grief, both redemptive and rebellious, fueled moral consciousness and humanitarian action rather than retaliation. They redirected their helplessness into advocacy soldiers at war overseas and for wounded warriors at home.

Combat Paper: mourning and materiality

Beyond the art practices I have used to work through difficult and/or traumatic experiences defying narrative representation, as a psychoanalyst I have explored the relational and reintegrative functions of art for those whose traumatic memory fragments can't be contained in words. Since the completion of my film, I have become a mental health support and research advisor for Combat Paper NJ, an affiliate of The Combat Paper Project, an organization that provides printmaking and hand papermaking workshops for veterans and their communities.

The philosophy and practice of Combat Paper originated when Drew Cameron, a veteran then-recently returned from Iraq, cut his uniform off his body and shredded, pulped, and pressed those fibers into handmade paper. He would go on to share the process with his peers, traveling across the country bringing workshops to veterans and their communities. Through Combat Paper, as the process viscerally enacts, the experience of mourning may be mediated through the body, which is temporarily displaced to the uniform.

Currently, groups of veterans are offered the opportunity to be taken from soldier to civilian–artist through this process of finding, reclaiming, reassembling, and enlivening fiber fragments of their military uniforms into handmade paper in the presence of a community of their peers. Combat Paper is made in many different settings, whether in veteran-only workshops, public gatherings, university classrooms, or individual artists' studios.

During a Combat Paper workshop veterans essentially perform the same ritual as Cameron, cutting up in the presence of a group of supportive peers his or her military uniform. This process is reminiscent of the ancient Jewish practice of Kriah, tearing one's clothing as a material expression of grief and anger following the death of a close loved one. This visceral affective discharge, a controlled act of anguish, rage, and destruction is performed in the presence of supportive family members. Tearing represents, on one level, the death itself that "tears" the loved one from the living, a violent act evoking the destructive force and the gravity of the experienced death. This practice assists in the activation of grief through sensory bodily-based memory, similar to the way Combat Paper participants often tear their uniforms apart, setting aside the scissors, an object for a more careful deconstruction of the uniform. In the act of tearing and cutting up a uniform, the violence within is transposed to an external act.

Donning a uniform is one of the first steps in becoming a member of the military and when they leave service veterans often take a duffle bag full of uniforms back to civilian life. While the uniform obscures personal identity it is also a bond of attachment to other soldiers. A military uniform is akin to a soldier's skin festooned with tattoos displaying eye-grabbing patches and campaign ribbons, a feisty advertisement of where this veteran has been. Once soaked in the dirt, sweat, and blood of war the material uniform fragments are, in a sense, "cleansed" in a water bath (the process of being "pulped" in a Hollander beater, a machine developed for macerating rags and fibers) and lastly pressed into sheets of handmade paper. The cleansing of the fragments may be seen as a process of purification of the simultaneously destructive and violated body held symbolically in the uniform.

This purification process reminds me of a similar practice of Rolling Thunder, Inc.: their monthly gathering to wash the Vietnam Veterans Memorial Wall, that physical object seen by many Vietnam veterans as symbolically holding the bodies of their lost comrades. These rituals are reminiscent of ancient cross-culture traditions, from the sweat lodges of Native Americans to the baths of the Vestal Virgins (French, 2003), designed to cleanse the returning soldier from the transgressions of combat in order to support their transition back to civilian life.

Combat Paper is not only a new surface, but also a symbolic container of reconstructed war experiences with the now-transformed and embedded material fragments of combat uniforms. While the resulting paper contains no explicit reference to any specific event, it embodies the veterans' military experience. This new surface, a container of symbolically reconstructed war experiences (though initially devoid of obvious visual representations or content), becomes a space (within the "safe space" created by the veterans in their workshop) upon which participants begin a process of self-witnessing, through printmaking and photographic transfer techniques. Veterans are "liberating the rag" in the sense that they are transforming a meaningful material into a new platform, freed of media, politics, and clichés, and derived from the transformative possibilities of their own creativity. The experience of war is held in these artworks, beyond the surface images, through enacting the subjective experience of mourning.

The well-known South African artist William Kentridge has described the process of making art as a form of slow-motion thinking, which over time, in its uncertain and imprecise fashion, constructs and serves as a model of *how* to construct meaning (Danto, 2007). In the interaction between implicit domain bodily gestures and art media, invisible memory becomes visible. In this process of forming, erasing, and modifying, emergent forms are captured and repossessed as they are "recognized" by the art maker as an equivalent of an "unthought-of thought" now seen and eventually known. The survivor artist begins to witness and dialogue with previously unrepresented aspects of the self in the construction of his or her own experience in the formation of the art product itself. This dialogue with their own traumatic subjective experience, now located in a viewable art product, holds many possibilities. After catastrophic loss, when the internal world is fractured—a state which often cannot be verbalized—the artmaking process pushes the subject to seek modes of expression of the unthought-of and/or of the unthinkable traumatic memory, co-creating aesthetic form in the interaction with materials, or discovered in pre-existing cultural aesthetic forms, that which resonates with his raw or sense memories.

The unique capacities of artmaking to capture, repossess, reintegrate and transmit dissociated emotional, sensory, or perceptual fragments, provides the experience(s) of trauma to be "known" and potentially supports the development from non-verbal expression to declarative meaning and creation of a meaningful and affectively rich narrative. Co-creating aesthetic and bodily-based sensory forms in the interaction with materials resonate with losses seeking representation. Through this process, one isn't just representing one's experience; rather, one's experience is being shaped in the process of representation with the attuned material as the self is encountered in the art object.

In the process of creating these relational aesthetic moments—between self and resonating art object, and eventually between self/art object and witnessing audience—memories can be re-embodied, or linked, with affects. Relational attachments, virtual or actual, can also be rebuilt, opening a dialogue with the world, mitigating isolation as the result of shame. Furthermore, the art product restores a sense of aliveness and integrative capacities for the maker.

By Our Own Hand: "It is in the shelter of each other that people live" (Irish Proverb)

This brings me to my current project, a public art installation I have designed as a containing space to facilitate and support community grieving, a collaboration between veterans and non-veteran organizers and artists around the country. Since the War on Terror began, 6,717 men and women have been killed in action according to the Department of Defense. During this time—and equally tragic—a larger and unknown number of US service members and veterans of these wars have died by their own hand.

I've conceived By Our Own Hand, a warehouse-scale art installation, as a response to not only those killed in action, but also to the soaring number of suicides among military personnel of the last decade. The installation is visually modeled after the ancient practice of Tibetan prayer flags hung to mark an important and challenging occasion where traditional wishes are

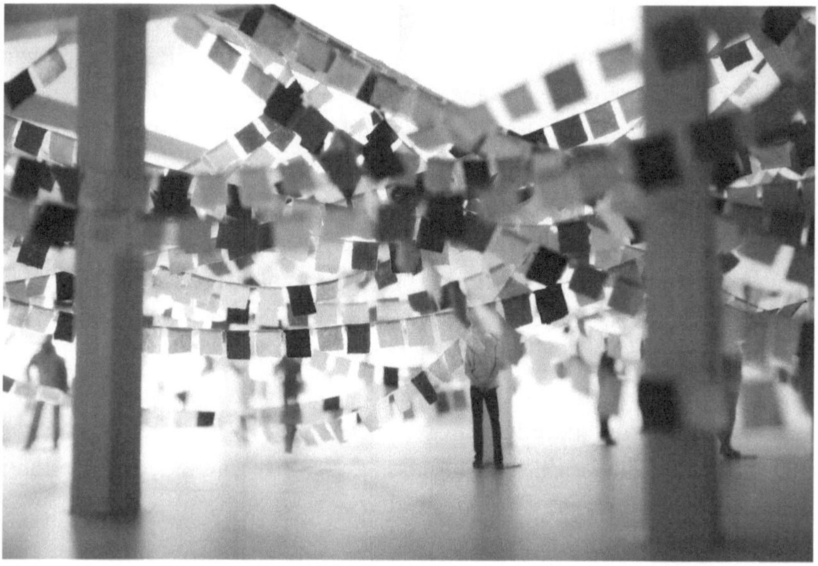

Figure 7.1 By Our Own Hand installation model.
Installation designed by Donna Bassin. Model by Robert Pyzocha. Photo by Steve Hellerstein, featured with his kind permission.

made for global peace, hope, strength, compassion, and protection from harm. For the installation, the flag-draped cords will attach to the ceiling and the walls at different heights to create a variety of visual planes, suggesting the weight and gravity of loss of life and producing an inner quiet within a contemplative space. In Tibetan tradition, it is believed that as the flags are shredded by the wind, the content within the flag will be released. Traditional belief suggests that even the slightest movement of the breeze will activate and release the prayers on the flags for the benefit of all. Ideally, the movement of the public walking through this space will activate the hanging flags, thus "releasing the prayers" associated with each. These paper flags of sacrificial remembrance will create a haunting canopy rising above a public space ideal for reflection and conversation. The enormity of the installation will make tangible the gravity of the rising death toll.

Sheets of Combat Paper, one for every killed in action, will be made at community workshops around the country. Each of the workshops will follow a structure designed to engage veteran and non-veteran communities, putting them in dialogue, sharing in the military experience by physically manipulating and reclaiming the "trace object," the military uniform. Current plans include the creation of an additional 22 sheets of combat paper to be made everyday at the installation. These will symbolically represent the 22 veteran suicides estimated to occur everyday. By Our Own Hand enlists the ethic of "leave no soldier behind" to attend to the epidemic rate of suicides among military personnel and veterans. It is hoped that critical reflection on the reasons for these self-inflicted deaths will result, thus unsettling a society largely apathetic to veteran issues.

Dynamic memorials such as the Vietnam Veterans Memorial or the recently constructed Reflecting Absence at the World Trade Center site, and the community's interaction with these aesthetically meaningful structures, constitute a dynamic memorialization process, providing opportunities for education, shared memory, and collective grieving. The actual material object—the wall, the fountains—are only one piece of the intersubjective collaboration. The public that is engaged and receptive to its power to elicit memory is the other piece.

Shay (1995) writes that when ancient Athenian warriors came home, the entire populace gathered at the foot of the Acropolis to accompany the warriors on a journey through mourning, reparation, and restitution. By Our Own Hand will provide such a gathering place for the general public, active duty service personnel, veterans, and their families in an attempt to recreate the respect and nurturing practices of ancient Athens toward returning warriors. The installation will invite the receptive viewer to enter in, experience, and explore along with the papermakers, promoting a mutual understanding of the consequences of the military experience, combat especially. This is an effort to create a space in which to remember and critically reflect (not necessarily to provide presence), encouraging the possibility of a more engaged remembrance. The idea of an Athenian chorus of citizens gathered at the Acropolis singing songs of purification to help restore moral integrity to those returning from war is a far cry from the rituals of modern American culture. In Ancient Greece, an entire populace wept and witnessed, accompanying the perpetrators of state-sponsored violence on their journey of mourning, helping warriors reintegrate back into society. Athenian tragedies, performed by combat veterans for an audience of returning warriors, were filled with violence and anguish and have been seen to be a form of civic group therapy (Meagher, 2006).

Veteran suicide is on the rise, yet remains a hushed subject in regard to how those fallen ought to be memorialized. Butler (2004, 2014) has written powerfully and extensively about the cultural refusal to mourn certain losses, those whose mourning is prohibited due to social stigma (e.g., the "ungrievable life" of an individual with AIDS, convicted criminals, drug addicts, and perhaps even suicides). She argues for public recognition of these losses. The perception of our military as heroes, victims or perpetrators, has led to a relative absence of community spaces where the losses of war might be named and mourned. A healthy society requires the creation of such spaces.

Toward a theory of collaborative mourning spaces: psychoanalytic perspectives applied to community

The creation of a collaborative mourning space, especially in a post-war context, calls on society (and the veteran) to perform the following:

First, one must find what has been lost and reawaken hidden grief. The narratives need to be found and told to a receptive other who serves as a witness. This includes a courageous acknowledgment of transgressions, an acceptance of responsibility and desire to make reparation for morally reprehensible acts during war. Stan Goff has said of his dehumanizing behavior during the war in Vietnam, "I can't take it back, I have to live with the consequences. But I can make amends" (Bassin, 2008, 2014).

Second, one must find a social structure to assist in the regulation of overwhelming affects and to validate the losses. Mourners can't grieve alone. Klein (1940) has suggested that bereavement requires the comfort of a good internal objector. However, as elaborated by Grand (2009), during trauma there is no sheltering parental body, no comforting parental presence, no containing parental mind to hold the overwhelming affects. As the (m)other originally bore witness to and helped organize the early effects of her infant, mourners require, as Hagman (2001) suggests, a community (or an other) to stand in for the mother, thus mourning with the mourner.

Third, a community of mourners should utilize the past as a generative medium for something new to emerge. Eigen (1999) has suggested that guilt and other psychic injury can be a way into deeper contact with ourselves and to the depths of others, into a deeper sense of life. Grief, for the veterans' communities I have worked within, was not marked under marble memorials or solemn ceremonies, but rather used to ignite attempts at restoration and reparation. They chose to use their pasts rather than suffer them.

Fourth, one must reconnect with the ethos of leave no soldier in one's civilian life and within one's community. In essence, what is needed is a re-establishment of the bonds of attachment, the relational ties that mitigate social isolation and promote self-forgiveness.

Lastly, organized protest and community actions should be used as a way to restore individual agency in a socio-political arena that is becoming evermore abstract and divisive. The process and "products" of the memorializing and protest activities discussed above assuage persecutory anxiety and survival guilt through restitution and reparation (Klein, 1937), highlighting Titchener's observations (1982) that the violent and destructive drives released during war must be attended to in order to treat "post-traumatic decline." Although the language differs, Bragin (2007/2010) has highlighted what the veterans intuitively understood: opportunities for reparation are necessary in the grieving process.

In the end, though, I've learned that one doesn't heal from war. One learns to surrender to the changes that loss brings. Butler (2014) speaks of mourning "… as a yielding to an unwanted transformation, where neither the full shape nor the import of that alteration can be known in advance." While the grief of others unsettles us, it allows us, according to Butler (2004), to experience vulnerability, thus enlarging the self through connection to the experience of others. In turn "bystanders" may transform into "good-enough" witnesses that may be moved to take ethical actions within their communities. Rosenbaum (2009) encourages us to consider the model of the legendary Greek poet and musician Orpheus who entered the bowels of the Underworld and returned as a task of the psychoanalyst working with survivors of violence. And while visionary architects of the socio-political implications of unresolved mourning such as Herman (1992/1997), Lifton (1993), Caruth (1996, 2014), Derrida (2001), Butler (2004), Laub (2005), and Boulanger (2007) have written theory and drawn philosophical blueprints for construction of an intersubjective ground in which traumatic losses can be processed, the details might best be found in the lives of those, such as combat veterans, who have created their own ways of working through collective traumas.

> And even though they said our war was over,
> It sure doesn't seem that way.
> But hopefully
> One of these days,
> We'll finally make it back home.

From "Game Over" (Wright, 2014)

Appendix

American Gold Star Mothers, Inc. is an organization of mothers who have lost a son or daughter in service to the United States. They are a Veterans Service Organization, established in 1928 and chartered by the US Congress in 1984. Nationally, the organization has approximately 2,000 members. www.goldstarmoms.org

Combat Paper Project hosts papermaking workshops, where veterans use their uniforms worn in service to create works of art. The uniforms are cut up, beaten into a pulp, and formed into sheets of paper. Participants use the transformative process of papermaking to reclaim their uniforms as art and express their experiences with the military. www.combatpaper.org

Iraq Veterans Against the War (IVAW) was formed in 2004. IVAW's membership includes recent veterans and active duty servicemen and women from all branches of military service, National Guard members, and reservists who have served in the US military since September 11, 2001. Since their inception, they have called for the immediate withdrawal of all occupying forces in Iraq; reparations for the human and structural damages Iraq has suffered; and full benefits, adequate healthcare (including mental health), and other support for returning servicemen and women. www.ivaw.org

Rolling Thunder, Inc. states their primary mission is to publicize the Prisoners of War–Missing in Action (POW–MIA) issue: to educate the public that many American Prisoners of War were left behind after all previous wars and to help correct the past and to protect the future veterans from being left behind should they become POW–MIA. While many members of Rolling Thunder, Inc. are veterans and many ride motorcycles, neither qualification is a prerequisite. www.rollingthunder1.com

Veterans for Peace (VFP) is comprised of over 140 chapters worldwide, whose work includes: educating the public on the consequences of militarism, advocating for a dismantling of the war economy, and providing services that assist veterans and victims of war. www.veteransforpeace.org

Vietnam Veterans Against the War (VVAW) was formed in 1967, and once boasted over 30,000 members. Throughout the 1970s, the organization worked to get PTSD officially recognized and advocated for veterans suffering agent orange exposure, while demonstrating publicly for the withdrawal of US troops from Indochina. They are still active today. www.vvaw.org

Warrior Writers' mission is to create a culture in which veterans and service members speak openly and honestly about their military experiences.

In the form of veteran-focused writing and artmaking workshops, participants are encouraged to share their stories in the form of books, performances, and exhibitions. They have released four anthologies of writing to date. www.warriorwriters.org

Notes

1 The veterans' poetry featured in this chapter is reprinted from *Warrior Writers: A Collection of Writing and Artwork by Veterans* (2014) with the kind permission of Kevin Basl and Warrior Writers.
2 See chapter appendix for detailed descriptions of organizations appearing herein.
3 The Wall is perceived as symbolically holding the bodies of those killed. The journey to the Wall and the interaction at the Wall, that is, the walk into its center (which implies seeing one's reflection in the black granite surface, and may include a search for the "body" of a lost soldier: finding a particular name, touching that name, and taking a rubbing as if reclaiming a piece of the deceased's body) is an attempt to find what has been lost.
4 Exposure to prolonged trauma and fear impacts on the brain's amygdala and hippocampus which not only regulate emotions but link emotions to memory.

References

Bassin, D. (Producer and Director). (2008, 2014). *Leave no soldier* [Motion picture]. USA: ShrinkWrap Productions.

Bouglanger, G. (2007). *Wounded by reality: Understanding and treating adult onset trauma*. London: The Analytic Press.

Bragin, M. (2007). Knowing terrible things: Engaging survivors of extreme violence in treatment. *Clinical Social Work Journal*, 35(4), 229–236.

Bragin, M. (2010). Can anyone here know who I am? Co-constructing meaningful narratives with combat veterans. *Clinical Social Work Journal*, 38(3), 316–326.

Butler, J. (2004). *Precarious life: The powers of mourning and violence*. London: Verso.

Butler, J. (2014, May 8). On the edge: Grief. Retrieved from www.pen.org/nonfiction/edge-grief, accessed November 20, 2015.

Carson, A. (2006). *Grief lesson: Four plays by Euripides*. New York: New York Review Books Classics.

Caruth, C. (1996). *Unclaimed experience: Trauma, narrative and history*. Baltimore: Johns Hopkins University Press.

Caruth, C. (2014). *Listening to trauma: Conversations with leaders in the theory and treatment of catastrophic experience*. Baltimore: Johns Hopkins University Press.

Danto, A. C. (2007). *Unnatural wonders: Essays from the gap between art and life*. New York: Columbia University Press.

Derrida, J. 2001. *On Cosmopolitanism and forgiveness*. Abingdon: Routledge.

Eigen, M. (1999). *Toxic nourishment*. London: Karnac Books.

Eng, D. L., and Kazanjian, D. (Eds). (2003). *Loss: The politics of mourning*. Berkeley: University of California Press.

French, S. E. (2003). *The code of the warrior: Exploring warrior values, past and present*. New York: Rowman and Littlefield Press.

Grand, S. (2009). *The hero in the mirror: From fear to fortitude*. London: Routledge.

Hagman, G. (2001). Beyond decathexis: Toward a new psychoanalytic understanding and treatment of mourning. In R. A. Neimeyer (Ed.), *Meaning reconstruction & the experience of loss* (pp. 13–31). Washington: American Psychological Association.

Herman, J. (1992, 1997). *Trauma and recovery: The aftermath of violence, from domestic abuse to political terror*. New York: Basic Books.

Klein, M. (1937, 1975). Love, guilt and reparation. In M. Klein (Ed.), *The writings of Melanie Klein, vol. I: Love, guilt and reparation and other works, 1921–1945* (pp. 306–344). New York: The Free Press.

Klein, M. (1940). Mourning and its relation to manic-depressive states. *The International Journal of Psychoanalysis*, 21, 125–153.

Laub, D. (2005) Traumatic shutdown of narrative and symbolization: A death instinct derivative? *Contemporary Psychoanalysis*, 41(2), 307–326.

Lifton R. J. (2005). *Home from the war: Learning from Vietnam veterans*. New York: Other Press.

Litz, B., Stein, N., Delaney, E., Lebowitz, L., Nash, W., Silva, C., and Maguen, S. (2009, December 9). Moral injury and moral repair in war veterans: A preliminary model and intervention strategy. *Clinical Psychology Review*, 29(8), 695–706.

Meagher, R. E. (2006). *Herakles gone mad: Rethinking heroism in an age of endless war*. Northampton: Olive Branch Press.

Morrison, T. (1987). *Beloved*. New York: Alfred A. Knopf, Inc.

O'Brien, T. (2009). *The things they carried*. Boston: Houghton Mifflin Harcourt.

Rosenbaum, R. (2009). Postponing trauma: The dangers of telling. *International Journal of Psychoanalysis*, 90(6), 1319–1340.

Segal, H. (1997). Silence is the real crime. In *Psychoanalysis, Literature and War* (pp. 143–156). London: Routledge.

Shay, J. (1994). *Achilles in Vietnam: Combat trauma and the undoing of character*. New York: Atheneum.

Shay, J. (1995). The birth of tragedy: Out of the needs of democracy. *Didaskalia: Ancient Theater Today,* 2(2). Retrieved from www.didaskalia.net/issues/vol2no2/shay.html, accessed November 18, 2015.

Shay, J. (2002). *Odysseus in American: Combat trauma and the trials of homecoming*. New York: Scribner.

Stainthorp Berggren, J. (2011). P.lease T.ry S.omething D.ifferent. In L. Calica (Ed.), *After action review: A collection of writing and artwork by veterans of the global war on terror* (pp. 144–147). Barre: Warrior Writers.

Titchener, J. (1982) Post-traumatic decline: A consequence of unresolved destructive drives. In Figley, C. (Ed.), *Trauma and its wake* (pp. 5–19). New York: Brunner/Mazel.

Turner, J. (2014). Standard operating procedure. In L. Calica and K. Basl (Eds), *Warrior writers: A collection of writing and artwork by veterans* (pp. 25–27). Barre: Warrior Writers.

Wright, E. (2014). Game over. In L. Calica and K. Basl (Eds), *Warrior writers: A collection of writing and artwork by veterans* (pp. 98–99). Barre: Warrior Writers.

Chapter 8

Large-group identity and massive trauma

Vamik D. Volkan

This chapter describes societal responses when the "Other," who possesses a different large-group identity than the victims, hurts, humiliates, and oppresses a large group and threatens its large group's identity. Large-group identities are articulated in terms of commonality such as "we are Basque; we are Lithuanian Jews; we are Ukrainian, we are Sunni Muslim; we are communist." Large-group identities are the end-result of myths and realities of common beginnings, historical continuities, geographical realities, and shared linguistic, societal, religious, cultural, and ideological factors. Belonging to a large group is a natural phenomenon in human life. Yet, a simple definition of large-group identity is not sufficient to explain the power it has to influence political, economic, legal, and military initiatives and to induce seemingly irrational resistances to finding peaceful solutions to large-group conflicts.

The canvas of a metaphorical tent

Think in terms of how we learn to wear two layers, like fabric, from the time we are children. The first layer, the individual layer, fits each of us snugly, like clothing. It is one's core personal identity that provides an inner sense of persistent sameness for the individual (Erikson, 1956). The second layer is like the canvas of a tent, which is loose fitting, but allows us to share a sense of sameness with others under the same large-group tent; it represents large-group identity. Some common threads, such as identifications with intimate others in one's childhood environment, are used in the construction of both layers. Thus, the individual identity and the large-group identity, psychologically speaking, are interconnected.

Under a huge large-group tent there are subgroups and subgroup identities, such as professional identities. My focus is not on such subgroups. In this chapter I will refer to large-group processes shared by the majority of persons under the metaphorical tent, leaving out certain people such as immigrants or those who may be products of parents from more than one ethnic or religious group. If a conflict erupts between two large groups, children who have parents who belong to two different ethnic or religious groups may, even as adults, have psychological problems. Furthermore, dissenters in a large group do not modify the basic elements of a large-group identity unless they have a huge following and thus they start an influential subgroup and become involved in a new large-group identity.

In our routine lives we are not keenly aware of our large-group identity, the canvas of the metaphorical tent, just as we are not usually aware of our constant breathing. If we have pneumonia or are in a burning building, we quickly notice each breath we take. Likewise, if the huge tent's canvas shakes or parts of it are torn apart by "Others," tens, hundreds of thousands, or millions of persons under the canvas become preoccupied with the canvas and will be emotionally ready to do anything to repair, maintain, and protect it, and when they do, they are often willing to tolerate extreme sadism or masochism if they think that what they are doing will help to maintain and protect their large-group identity (Volkan, 1988, 1997, 2004, 2006a, 2013, 2014a).

Each large-group identity includes tribal, ethnic, national, religious, or ideological "identity markers" that only belong to its members. We can visualize different colorful designs that are stitched on the canvas of each large group's metaphorical tent. These designs are related to physical body characteristics, language, nursery rhymes, food, dances, religious beliefs, myths, flags, geographical investments, heroes, martyrs, and images of historical events. They only belong and are meaningful to tens, hundreds of thousands, or millions of people living under the same metaphorical tent. On occasion, a design on a canvas, such as a certain religious element, may appear similar to a design on another huge tent's canvas. However, even under these circumstances we usually note "minor differences" in such elements (Horowitz, 1985; Volkan, 1997, 2013, 2014a). When conflicts arise between the two large groups, such minor differences become major concerns.

Chosen glories and chosen traumas

Two types of design on the metaphorical tent's canvas represent some specific realistic and/or mythologized past historical events and heroes and martyrs associated with them. Such historical events can be categorized as glorified or traumatic; usually they are both. In 1999 I described the terms "chosen glory" and "chosen trauma" for the first time. Chosen glories are shared mental representations of pride and pleasure evoking past events and heroes that are recollected ritualistically. Past victories in battle and great accomplishments of a political or religious nature frequently appear as chosen glories. For example, large groups celebrate their independence days.

Chosen glories are passed on to succeeding generations in parent/teacher–child interactions and through participation in ritualistic ceremonies. They link children of a large group with each other and the children experience increased self-esteem by being associated with such glories. In stressful situations political leaders reactivate the mental representations of chosen glories and heroes associated with them to bolster the shared identity of their followers. During the first Gulf War Saddam Hussein made many references to Sultan Saladin's victories over the Crusaders, even though Saladin was not an Arab, but a Kurd.

A chosen trauma is the shared mental representation of a massive trauma in a large group's history in which the group suffered catastrophic loss, humiliation, and helplessness at the hands of its enemies. While chosen glories increase collective self-esteem, they do not burden the next generation(s) with complicated shared psychological tasks as chosen traumas do. Below I will explain such tasks and illustrate why chosen traumas, in supporting large-group identity and its cohesiveness, are more complex than chosen glories and why chosen traumas are much stronger large-group identity markers than chosen glories. However, sometimes chosen traumas and chosen glories appear as intertwined.

Massive traumas at the hand of the "Other"

Large groups' massive traumas are of various types. Some are from natural causes, such as tropical storms, floods, volcanic eruptions, forest fires, or earthquakes. Some societal traumas are accidental man-made disasters, like the 1986 Chernobyl accident that spewed tons of radioactive dust into the atmosphere. Sometimes, the death of a person who functioned as a shared "transference figure" for many members of the large group provokes traumatic societal responses—as did the assassinations of John F. Kennedy (Wofenstein and Kliman, 1965) and Martin Luther King, Jr. in the United States, Yitzhak Rabin in Israel (Erlich, 1998; Raviv, Sadeh, Raviv, Silberstein and Diver, 2000; Moses-Hrushovski, 2000), Prime Minister Olof Palme in Sweden, the National Democratic Party leader Giorgi Chanturia in the Republic of Georgia, former Prime Minister Rafik Hariri in Lebanon or the deaths of the American astronauts, especially teacher Christa McAuliffe, in the 1986 space shuttle Challenger explosion (Volkan, 1997). Other massive traumas are due to the deliberate actions of an enemy group, as in ethnic, national, religious, and political ideological conflicts. Such catastrophes themselves range from chronic mistreatment or oppression of a group by the "Other" within one national boundary, to terrorist attacks, wars, and even genocide, and from the traumatized group actively fighting its powerful enemy in desperation to the traumatized group being rendered completely passive and helpless.

When nature shows its fury and people suffer, those affected tend ultimately to accept the event as fate or as the will of God (Lifton and Olson, 1976). Following man-made accidental disasters, survivors blame a small number of individuals or governmental organizations for their carelessness. When a leader is killed (not by the "Other" but by an individual belonging to the same large group as did the leader) the rage is against that killer and, if one exists, against the political organization to which the killer belongs. However, when a trauma results from oppression, war, or other ethnic, national, religious, or ideological conflict, especially when the victimized large group is rendered passive and helpless, there is an identifiable enemy large group that has deliberately inflicted pain, humiliation, environmental restriction, destruction, and death on its victims. Such collective trauma takes place because the affected large group and the perpetrators belong to different large groups and the killing and the destruction is in the name of large-group identity (Volkan, 1997, 2013, 2014a). Only this kind of trauma may evolve as a chosen trauma. A large group does not "choose" to be victimized by another large group and subsequently lose self-esteem, but it does "choose" to psychologize and dwell on a past traumatic event and make it a major design to be stitched on the canvas of a large-group tent.

After a massive trauma at the hands of the "Other," members of a large group will face difficult tasks taming and rendering harmless the following psychological features:

1 sense of victimization and exposure to dehumanization;
2 sense of pain and open or hidden humiliation due to helplessness;
3 sense of guilt for surviving while others perished;
4 difficulty being assertive without facing humiliation;
5 increase in externalizations/projections and thus exaggeration of "bad" prejudice;
6 increase in narcissistic investment in large-group identity;
7 envy toward the victimizer and (defensive) identification with the oppressor;
8 difficulty, or often inability, to mourn losses.

When such shared psychological experiences continue and the members of a large group cannot find adaptive solutions for them, they become involved in the next shared experience:

9 shared transgenerational transmission of psychological tasks to deal with the influence of the trauma.

Meanwhile the perpetrators will experience shame and guilt (may be hidden) for hurting others and such shared emotions too are involved in transgenerational transmissions. Collective transgenerational transmissions lead to the establishment of chosen traumas.

Transgenerational transmissions

Knowledge of transgenerational transmissions of trauma from one generation to the next mainly comes from studies on Jewish people who were survivors of the Holocaust and their offspring. The literature on this topic is vast. (For information on such studies see: Grubrich-Simitis, 1979; Kestenberg and Brenner, 1996; Volkan, Ast and Greer, 2002; Brenner, 2004; and Fromm, 2012). Here I will first describe briefly how transgenerational transmission occurs between an adult and a developing child and second how collective transgenerational transmission takes place.

There is fluidity between a child's "psychic borders" and those of the mother and other caretakers, and the child–mother/caretaker experiences generally function as a kind of "incubator" for the child's developing mind.

Besides growth-initiating elements, however, the caretaker from the older generation can also transmit undesirable psychological elements to the child. One of the best-known examples of a relatively simple negative form of transgenerational transmission comes from Anna Freud and Dorothy Burlingham's observations of women and children during the Nazi attacks on London. Anna Freud and Dorothy Burlingham (1942) noted that small children under the age of three did not become anxious during the bombings unless their mothers were afraid. The fluidity mentioned above also may occur among adults under certain conditions of regression, such as during and after massive catastrophes at the hand of others.

There are many forms of transgenerational transmission. Besides anxiety, depression, elation, worries, and fantasies, there are various psychological tasks that an adult may assign to a child. I will now describe a concept which I call "depositing" (Volkan, 2006a, 2013, 2014a; Volkan, Ast, Greer, 2002) and its role in transgenerational transmissions. In the well-known psychological process called identification, children are the primary active actors in collecting images and tasks from their environment and making these images and tasks their own. In depositing it is the adult in the child's environment who has a psychological urgency to put something, an image associated with certain psychological tasks, into the developing child's psyche. This process fits well to Melanie Klein's (1946) description of "projective identification." However, since I am describing the creation of a kind of "psychological DNA" within the child, a foundation for his or her identity formation, I prefer to use the term "depositing" and differentiating this term from projective identification in everyday use. Anne Ancelin Schützenberger's (1998) "ancestor syndrome," Judith Kestenberg's term (1982) "transgenerational transposition," and Haydée Faimberg's (2005) description of "the telescoping of generations" refer to depositing traumatized images; however these authors do not describe clearly how this process takes place.

An adult may "deposit" his or her own injured self-images within the child along with images of others who were involved in the traumatic event—even sometimes the image of the perpetrator—and then give psychological tasks to these transferred images that aim to ease the pain and terror of the original trauma or control the outcome of the trauma. The experiences that created these mental images in the adult are not accessible to the child; yet, those mental images are pushed into the child, without the experiential/contextual framework that created them. Memories belonging to one person cannot be transmitted to another person, but an adult can deposit his or her traumatized self and other images into a child's self-representation and assign tasks to such internal images (Volkan, 2006a; Volkan, Ast and Greer, 2002). When Peter was a very small child his biological father abandoned him. A man who would be his stepfather entered into his life and "saved" him from a smothering, humiliating home environment. Peter's stepfather was a survivor of the 1942 Bataan Death March and Japanese war camps in the Philippines. He deposited his self-representation, severely traumatized during the Second World War, into the developing self-representation of little Peter and gave him a task to be a vicious hunter instead of being hunted. Peter had a prestigious job in the American weapons industry. But, when he faced a humiliating event, such as feeling rejected by his wife or losing a competition in his work situation, he needed to kill animals. He would fly in a helicopter over a herd of deer and machine gun the animals and watch their bellies explode (Volkan, 2014b).

Collective transgenerational transmissions

After experiencing a collective catastrophe inflicted by an enemy large group, affected individuals are left with self-images similarly (though not identically) traumatized by the shared event. Tens, hundreds of thousands, or millions of individuals deposit such images into their children and give them tasks such as: "Regain my self-esteem for me," "Put my mourning process on the right tract," or "Be assertive and take revenge." It is this transgenerational conveyance of long-term "tasks" that perpetuate the cycle of societal trauma. Though each child in the second generation has his or her own individualized personality, all share similar links to the trauma's mental representation and similar unconscious tasks for coping with that representation. If the next generation cannot effectively fulfill their shared tasks—and this is usually the case—they will pass these tasks on to the third generation, and so on. Such conditions create a powerful unseen network among tens, hundreds of thousands, or millions of people.

Depending on external conditions, shared tasks may change from generation to generation. For example, in one generation the shared task may be to grieve the ancestors' loss and to feel their victimization. In the following generation, the shared task may be to express a sense of revenge for that loss and victimization. But whatever its expression in a given generation, keeping alive the mental representation of the ancestors' trauma remains the core task. As decades pass, the mental image of the ancestors' historical event, with references to heroes and martyrs, continues to link all the individuals in the large group. For the new generations, the meaning of the above tasks go through change of function (Waelder, 1930); now the mental image of the event is used to link all members of the large group together. When an ancestors' massive trauma takes this course the shared mental image of the ancestors' trauma involves a chosen trauma—chosen to become a most significant large-group identity marker (Volkan, 1988, 1997, 2004, 2006a, 2013, 2014a). Similar processes may also appear in the descendants of victimizers. Among the descendants of perpetrators there is more preoccupation with consequences of shared feelings of guilt than preoccupation with the shared feeling of humiliation. Both groups share a difficulty or inability to mourn (Mitscherlich and Mitscherlich, 1975).

Not all past massive tragedies at the hands of others evolve as chosen traumas. The mythologizing of victimized heroes and telling of moving stories associated with a collective trauma popularized in songs and poetry, and political leaders of later times creating a preoccupation with a past trauma and related events, play a role in turning a historic event into a chosen trauma. There are firmly established chosen traumas: Russians recall the "memory" of the Tatar-Mongol invasions in the thirteenth and fourteenth centuries; Greeks link themselves when they share the "memory" of the fall of Constantinople (Istanbul) to the Turks in 1453; Czechs commemorate the 1620 Battle of Bila Hora, which led to their subjugation under the Hapsburg Empire for nearly 300 years; Scots keep alive the story of the battle of Culloden of 1746 and the failure of Bonnie Prince Charlie to restore a Stuart to the British throne; the Dakota people of the United States recall the anniversary of their decimation at Wounded Knee in 1890; Crimean Tatars define themselves by their collective suffering during their deportation from Crimea in 1944; Israelis and Jews around the globe, including those not personally affected by the Holocaust, all define their large-group identity by direct or indirect references to it. The Holocaust is still too "hot" to be considered a truly established chosen trauma as described above, but it already has become a large-group marker, even though Orthodox Jews still refer to the 586 BC destruction of the Jewish temple in Jerusalem by Nebuchadnezzar II of Babylonia as the chosen trauma of the Jews. Some chosen traumas are difficult to detect because they are not simply connected to one well-recognized historical event. For example, the Estonians' chosen trauma seems unrelated to one specific event, but to the fact that they had lived under almost constant dominance (Swedes, Germans, Russians) for thousands of years.

For Shiites, the Battle of Karbala that took place in 680 (the year 61 of the Islamic calendar) in present-day Iraq has the most significant place in their religious large-group identity. It was during this battle that Husain, a son of the fourth Caliph Ali ibn Abi Talip and grandson of the Prophet Mohammed, together with his family and followers, were deprived of water and killed upon the desert plain by soldiers of Yezid, the claimant of the caliphate. Shiites believe that after the death of Mohamed in 632, religious leadership of the Islamic faith belonged to Ali ibn Abi Talip, Husain's father. Ali was passed over, however and, when he was finally proclaimed caliph, his rule was opposed by Mu'awiyah ibn Sufyan. Ali was succeeded by his son Hasan, who Shiites believe was poisoned at the behest of Mu'awiyah, who then became caliph. Husain reportedly refused to pledge his allegiance to him, and was attempting to lead his family to safety when he was attacked by Mu'awiyah's son Yezid in Karbala. As a chosen trauma, Shiites relive this historical atrocity on the anniversary of the Karbala Battle. Those Westerners who are interested in present-day Iran's internal and external affairs need to study the psychological influence this Shiite chosen trauma has on the Iranian large group's social, cultural, and political processes.

Entitlement ideologies

Affective aspects of some chosen traumas may remain dormant, and some chosen traumas may only be recalled during anniversaries. However, those that become connected with what I term "entitlement ideologies" (Volkan, 2006a, 2013) are prone to reactivation by emotions, and play a significant role in large-group social, political, and military affairs. Entitlement ideologies refer to a shared sense of entitlement to recover what was lost in reality and fantasy during the collective trauma that evolved as a chosen trauma and during other related shared traumas. Or they refer to the mythologized birth of a large group, a process that later generations idealize. They deny difficulties and losses that had occurred during it, and imagine their large group as if it is composed of persons belonging to a superior species. Holding on to an entitlement ideology primarily reflects a complication in large-group mourning, an attempt both to deny losses as well as a wish to recover them, a narcissistic reorganization accompanied by "bad" prejudice for the other.

Each large group's entitlement ideology is specific. Some entitlement ideologies are known by specific names in the literature. What Italians call "irredentism" (related to Italia Irredenta), what Greeks call "Megali Idea" (Great Idea), what Turks call "Pan-Turanism," what Serbs call "Christoslavism," and what extreme religious Islamists of today call "the return of an Islamic Empire" are examples of entitlement ideologies. Nancy Hollander (2010) describes how the American entitlement ideology, usually called "American exceptionalism," was inflamed after September 11, 2001. Such ideologies may last for centuries and may disappear and reappear when historical circumstances change and chosen traumas are activated. They contaminate diplomatic negotiations. They may result in changing the world map in peaceful or, unfortunately too often, dreadful ways.

An example of reactivation of a chosen trauma and an entitlement ideology

A chosen trauma that I studied in depth (Volkan, 1997) is the Serbian chosen trauma, the shared mental representation of the Battle of Kosovo in 1389, along with the entitlement ideology Christoslavism (Sells, 2002) to which it is linked. I believe that this is critical to understanding the contributions of large-group psychology in the tragedies in Bosnia in 1992 and in Kosovo in 1999. Despite the fact that in 1389 the leaders of both sides—Ottoman Sultan Murat I and Serbian Prince Lazar—were both killed during the Battle of Kosovo, and despite the fact that Serbia remained autonomous for over 70 years after the battle, the shared representation of the battle evolved as the major Serbian chosen trauma, marking the end of a glorious period of Serbian power and the beginning of their subjugation to the Ottoman Empire. In certain periods, Prince Lazar's image was used to cement a shared sense of victimization and martyrdom under Muslim rule; during others, his image became a symbol of the Serbs' desire to reverse the humiliation of the loss by reconquering Kosovo. As decades passed, Prince Lazar became associated with Jesus Christ, and icons showing Lazar's representation in fact decorated many Serbian churches throughout the six centuries following the battle. Even after Kosovo Province was taken back from the Ottoman Turks in the late nineteenth century, Lazar's "ghost" was still not put to rest. During the communist period when the government discouraged hero worship, Serbs were able to drink (introject) a popular red wine called "Prince Lazar."

After the collapse of communism, mental representations of Lazar and the Battle of Kosovo were resurrected by Slobodan Milošević, along with some members of the Serbian church and some members of the Serbian academic community. As the six-hundredth anniversary of the Battle of Kosovo approached in 1989, with the permission and encouragement of Milošević, Lazar's 600-year-old remains, which had been kept north of Belgrade, were placed in a coffin and taken, over the course of the year, to almost every Serb village and town, where they were received by huge crowds of mourners dressed in black. Again and again during this long journey, Lazar's remains were symbolically buried and reincarnated, until they were buried for good at the original battleground in Kosovo on June 28, 1989. The Serbian people began feeling, without being aware of it, that the defeat at the Battle of Kosovo had occurred only recently, a development made possible by the fact that the chosen trauma had been kept effectively alive for centuries.

On June 28, 1989, the six-hundredth anniversary of the Battle of Kosovo, a helicopter brought Serbian President Slobodan Milošević to the burial ground where a huge monument made of red stone symbolizing blood had been built. In the mythology, Prince Lazar had chosen the Kingdom of Heaven over the Kingdom of Earth. By design, Milošević descended from a helicopter, representing Prince Lazar/Jesus Christ coming to earth to find a new Kingdom, a Greater Serbia. Propaganda prepared an atmosphere that allowed the inflammation of the Serbian entitlement ideology, Christoslavism (Sells, 2002), which gave permission to create a Greater Serbia. Atrocities would eventually be committed against Bosnian and Kosovar Muslims, whom modern Serbs came to perceive as extensions of the Ottoman enemy of distant history. Thus, the Serbian large-group identity was reinforced and reinvigorated by the lasting emotional power of this ancient event—at terrible cost to non-Serbs.

Time collapse

Reactivated chosen trauma and entitlement ideology strengthen the people's sense of belonging to the same group, their shared large-group identity. Their reactivation may become a crucial resistance to finding a peaceful solution to the group's problems involving its current enemies.

Even though a chosen trauma refers to ancestors' victimhood, the current group does not wish to give up its investment in it. To do so would mean giving up a significant aspect of the shared large-group identity, so the large group resists making peace with its contemporary enemy.

Reactivation of a large group's chosen trauma and an entitlement ideology linked to it lead to "time collapse." Feelings, thoughts, wishes, and fears stimulated by the shared reactivation of the chosen trauma and the entitlement ideology collapse into perceptions and affects about a current international conflict and magnified dangers. When Slobodan Milošević and his associates reactivated the Serbian chosen trauma and the Serbian entitlement ideology it created a time collapse that led to genocidal acts in Europe at the end of the twentieth century. What can be done to promote peaceful co-existence between former "enemy" large groups?

Expressions of apology and forgiveness should not be considered as having magical diplomatic and political consequences. Some such apologies were experienced as genuine, while others were perceived as empty gestures. Furthermore, the concepts of apology and forgiveness cannot be fully understood without considering involuntary human conditions: mourning over losing people, possessions, land, prestige, honor, and so on. The mourning process means going over the images of lost persons and things, with associated feelings, hundreds of times until the reality of the loss is genuinely accepted and emotions—ranging from sadness to fury to survival guilt—are tamed. Forgiveness and societal well-being will be possible when societal mourning takes place or is tamed and "mental representations" of lost persons and things become futureless (Tähkä, 1984) but valued memories.

Arts, movies, poems, seminars, or conferences help to open the societal mourning process

Another typical way that a large group deals with mourning is to build monuments or memorials related to the massive trauma or to their ancestors' massive trauma at the hands of others. Some monuments are designed to keep wounds open. Others help the traumatized society to mourn (Volkan, 2006b).

My colleagues and I from the University of Virginia's Center for the Study of Mind and Human Interaction (CSMHI) (closed in 2005) developed strategies for peaceful co-existence between former "enemy" large groups. We named our methodology the Tree Model and I described it in detail previously (Volkan, 1999, 2013). The root, trunk, and branches of a tree represent the three phases of this model.

During the first phase, which includes in-depth psychoanalytically informed interviews with a wide range of the two opposing large groups' members, the facilitating team (composed of psychoanalysts, historians, political scientists, others from different disciplines and former high-level diplomats) begins to understand the main conscious as well as unconscious aspects of the relationship between opposing large groups and the surrounding situation to be addressed.

During the second phase, psychopolitical dialogues between the same 15 to 20 influential representatives (legislators, ambassadors, government officials, well-known scholars, or other public figures) of opposing large groups under the direction of the psychoanalytically informed facilitating team take place in a series of multi-day meetings over several years. The dialogue participants from the opposing groups are usually identified and selected during the diagnostic period. Although the capacity of participants to influence others outside the dialogue group will ultimately determine the impact of the process on the community at large, CSMHI found that it can be counterproductive to include top political leaders. Often it is members of the next level down in government who make the most suitable participants, since they can be freer from political pressures and more able to change their own attitudes, yet still influential. These participants become more effective negotiators of their large-group conflicts when the facilitators help them to hold on to "their individuality and began seeing those in the other group also as separate and distinct individuals … in some ways like themselves, with similar feelings, aspirations, fears and shortcomings" (Volkan, 2013, p. 42). This "psychological understanding" of others, when overlooked, effectively insures the failure of negotiations.

There are plenary sessions, but most of the work is done in small groups led by members of the facilitating team. The participants from the opposing large groups become spokespersons for their tribal, ethnic, national, religious, or ideological large groups. When two large groups are in conflict, the enemy is obviously real, but it is also fantasized. If participants can differentiate their fantasized dangers from the current issues, then negotiations and steps toward peace can become more realistic. Psychopolitical dialogues become a process in which historical grievances are aired; perceptions, fears, and attitudes are articulated; and previously hidden psychological obstacles to reconciliation or change rise to the surface. Their aim is not to erase the images of past historical events and differences in large-group identity and culture, but rather to detoxify the relationship so that differences do not lead to renewed violence.

Political and diplomatic efforts to find peaceful co-existence between enemies provoke shared, felt, or hidden anxiety, and therefore shared psychological obstacles against peaceful solutions because they threaten existing large-group identities, despite the fact that at times the population may appear to favor such changes. As a way of handling the opposing large groups' anxiety, the facilitating team pays attention to two basic principles that govern the interactions between enemies in acute conflict:

1. two opposing large groups need to maintain their identities as distinct from each other (principle of non-sameness) and;
2. two opposing large groups need to maintain an unambiguous psychological border between them. If a political border exists between the enemies, it becomes highly psychological.

Both principles relate to the fact that people in one large group have a tendency to externalize, project, and displace certain unwanted elements onto the other. Imagine "mud" is thrown onto the "Other's" huge metaphorical tent's canvas, and it sometimes leaves a "stain." There is, however, also anxiety that the "mud" could be hurled right back at the sender. The two principles exist to prevent the "mud" from coming back, thus helping each side's identity remain cohesive.

The act of paying attention to differences, including minor ones, between two large groups in conflict can be seen as a way of shoring up the psychological border between the two large groups' identities. This differentiation helps lessen each group's anxiety, since, with the psychological border in place, a clear distinction between the two large groups is maintained, diminishing the anxiety that one large group's identity will become diluted or lost in the "Other's" identity. This emphasis differentiates this facilitating team's strategy from many other peacemaking persons' or teams' insistence that in order to make peace the opposing groups are required to be friendly and that enemies need to "love" each other in order to make peace.

During psychopolitical dialogues the participants from the opposing large groups may suddenly experience a rapprochement. This closeness is then followed by a sudden withdrawal from one another and then again by closeness—coming together and then pulling apart like an accordion. Denying and accepting derivatives of aggression within the participants toward the "enemy" large group, even when they are hidden, and attempts to protect large-group identities underlie this behavior. Effective discussion of real-world issues cannot take place unless one allows the "accordion playing" to continue for a while so that the swing in sentiments can be replaced by more secure feelings about participants' large-group identities.

It will be sufficient to state that during the psychopolitical dialogues, the facilitating team pays full attention to large-group issues mentioned earlier in this chapter. It takes into consideration the importance of threats against large-group identity, it notices the importance of the shared mental representations of the large groups' histories, and includes the impact of transgenerational transmission of trauma, chosen traumas, entitlement ideologies as well as time collapse. One crucial aim of the psychopolitical dialogues is to establish a time expansion between the more recent problems and the past ones belonging to the ancestors so that more realistic negotiations about current issues can take place. This is done by not forgetting or denying ancestors' traumas, but by understanding and feeling how the mental representations of such traumas have become large-group identity markers.

The maturity and success of the facilitating team's approach will depend on clearly defining their task, developing a working alliance among themselves, and having a nonregressed relationship with their leader. Thus, it is important that the neutral team work together for some time before convening the dialogues in order to develop into a work group and to have a good grasp of the issues involved between the parties. Frequent debriefing among facilitating team members is essential during the psychopolitical dialogues. At the end of each day, CSMHI team members met to share their observations and work through potential difficulties they might be experiencing. Some facilitators may favor one antagonist group over the other. Like the participants, they may develop transference and countertransference attitudes toward particular participants or toward political leaders who are not in the room. Participants, on the other hand, may develop unrealistic fantasized expectations of the facilitators. During their nightly meetings, the facilitating team should discuss and work through such issues together.

The facilitating team seeks to spread the insights gained to the broader population through concrete programs that promote peaceful strategies and co-existence. In order for the gained insights to have an impact on social and political policy as well as on the populace at large, the final phase requires the collaborative development of concrete actions, programs, legal changes, and institutions. What is learned is operationalized so that more peaceful co-existence can be achieved.

Last comments

Besides the issues that are originally connected with chosen traumas and their reactivations, other specific psychological processes are present within any large group. These processes, such as circumstances that increase the need to have enemies, shared transference expectations from a political leader, a political leader's utilization of the large-group arena for finding solutions for personal conflicts, also require formulations. Because of the reality that many factors in large-group psychology stand side by side and complicate the existing realistic situation, any attempt to understand large groups may be very difficult and even impossible (Shapiro and Carr, 2006). But, I have become convinced that our developing a large-group psychology in its own right has a contribution to make.

What does large-group psychology in its own right mean? There are echoes of individual psychology in large-group psychology shared by tens, hundreds of thousands, or millions of persons, but large groups do not have one brain to think with or two eyes to cry. The multitudes of people in a large group share a psychological journey, such as complicated mourning after major shared losses at the hand of the "Other." Such journeys become sustained social, cultural, political, or ideological processes that are specific for the large group under study. Considering large-group psychology in its own right means making formulations as to a large groups' conscious and unconscious shared psychological experiences and motivations that initiate specific social, cultural, political, or ideological processes that influence this large group's internal and external affairs. I hope that psychoanalysts, group analysts, and psychoanalytically oriented clinicians will continue to develop large-group psychology in its own right, become involved in interdisciplinary initiatives, provide information on large-group identity and related concepts that can be used by diplomats and other authorities and make efforts for large groups' psychological well-being.

References

Brenner, I. 2004. *Psychic Trauma: Dynamics, Symptoms, and Treatment.* New York: Jason Aronson.

Erikson, E. H. 1956. The problem of ego identity. *Journal of the American Psychoanalytic Association*, 4:56–121.

Erlich, H. S. 1998. Adolescents' reactions to Rabin's assassination: A case of patricide? In *Adolescent Psychiatry: Developmental and Clinical Studies*, ed. A. Esman, pp. 189–205. London: The Analytic Press.

Faimberg, H. 2005. *The Telescoping of Generations. Listening to the Narcissistic Links Between Generations.* London: Routledge.

Freud, A. and Burlingham, D. 1942. *War and Children.* New York: International Universities Press.

Fromm, M. G. 2012 (Ed.). *Lost in Transmission: Studies of Trauma Across Generations.* London: Karnac.

Grubrich-Simitis, I. (1979). Extremtraumatisierung als kumulatives Trauma. Psychoanalytische Studien über seelische Nachwirkungen der Konzentrationslagerhaft bei Überlebenden und ihren Kindern (Extreme traumatization as a cumulative trauma. Psychoanalytic studies on the mental effects of imprisonment in concentration camps on survivors and their children). *Psyche,* 33:991–1023.

Hollander, N. 2010. *Uprooted Minds: Surviving the Political Terror in the Americas.* New York: Taylor and Francis.

Horowitz, D. L. 1985. *Ethnic Groups in Conflict.* Berkeley: University of California Press.

Kestenberg, J. S. 1982. A psychological assessment based on analysis of a survivor's child. In *Generations of the Holocaust*, eds M. S. Bergman and M. E. Jucovy, pp. 158–177. New York: Columbia University Press.

Kestenberg, J. S. and Brenner, I. 1996. *The Last Witness: The Child Survivor of the Holocaust.* Washington, DC: American Psychiatric Press.

Klein, M. 1946. Notes on some schizoid mechanisms. In *Development of Psychoanalysis*, ed. J. Riviere, pp. 292–320. London: Hogarth Press.

Lifton, R. and Olson, E. 1976. The human meaning of total disaster: The Buffalo Creek experience. *Psychiatry*, 39:1–18.

Mitscherlich, A. and Mitscherlich, M. 1975. *The Inability to Mourn: Principles of Collective Behavior.* Trans. B. R. Placzek. New York: Grove Press (1967).

Moses-Hrushovski, R. 2000. *Grief and Grievance: The Assassination of Yitzhak Rabin.* London: Minerva Press.

Raviv, A., Sadeh, A., Raviv, A., Silberstein, O., and Diver, O. 2000. Young Israelis' reactions to national trauma: The Rabin assassination and terror attacks. *Political Psychology*, 21:299–322.

Schützenberger, A. A. (1998). *The Ancestor Syndrome: Transgenerational Psychotherapy and the Hidden Links in the Family Tree.* New York: Routledge.

Sells, M. A. 2002. The construction of Islam in Serbian religious mythology and its consequences. In *Islam and Bosnia.* ed. M. Shatzmiller, pp. 56–85. Montreal: McGill University Press.

Shapiro, E. and Carr, W. 2006. Those people were some kind of solution: Can society in any sense be understood? *Organizational & Social Dynamics*, 6:241–257.

Tähkä, V. 1984. Dealing with object loss. *Scandinavian Psychoanalytic Review*, 7:13–33.

Volkan, V. D. 1988. *The Need to Have Enemies and Allies: From Clinical Practice to International Relationships.* Northvale: Jason Aronson.

Volkan, V. D. 1997. *Bloodlines: From Ethnic Pride to Ethnic Terrorism.* New York: Farrar, Straus and Giroux.

Volkan, V. D. 1999. The Tree Model: A comprehensive psychopolitical approach to unofficial diplomacy and the reduction of tension. *Mind and Human Interaction*, 10:142–210.

Volkan, V. D. 2004. *Blind Trust: Large Groups and Their Leaders in Times of Crises and Terror.* Charlottesville: Pitchstone Publishing.

Volkan, V. D. 2006a. *Killing in the Name of Identity: A Study of Bloody Conflicts.* Charlottesville: Pitchstone Publishing.

Volkan, V. D. 2006b. What some monuments tell us about mourning and forgiveness. In *Taking Wrongs Seriously: Apologies and Reconciliation*, eds E. Barkin and A. Karn, pp. 115–131. Stanford: Stanford University Press.

Volkan, V. D. 2013. *Enemies on the Couch: A Psychopolitical Journey through War and Peace.* Durham: Pitchstone.

Volkan, V. D. 2014a. *Psychoanalysis, International Relations, and Diplomacy: A Sourcebook on Large-Group Psychology.* London: Karnac.

Volkan, V. D. 2014b. *Animal Killer: Transmission of War Trauma from One Generation to the Next.* London: Karnac.

Volkan, V. D., Ast, G. and Greer, W. 2002. *The Third Reich in the Unconscious: Transgenerational Transmission and its Consequences.* New York: Brunner-Routledge.

Waelder, R. (1930). The principle of multiple function: Observations on overdetermination. *Psychoanalytic Quarterly*, 5:45–62 (1936).

Wolfenstein, M. and Kliman, G. (eds) 1965. *Children and the Death of a President: Multi-disciplinary Studies.* Garden City: Doubleday.

Part IV

Psychoanalytic scholarship and activism

Chapter 9

The analyst as witness, historian and activist

A conversation with Robert Jay Lifton[1]

Elizabeth R. Goren and Judith L. Alpert

Introduction

We had the honor of interviewing Dr. Robert Jay Lifton in his New York City home on April 15, 2012. Given space limitations, we cannot include the entire transcript of the one and one-half hour interview. However, we are delighted to include parts of this interview here. While we exercised editorial privilege in transcribing the interview, Dr. Lifton approved all the edits and none of the edits altered the intended meaning. Our interview focused on his noted professional work as a psychoanalytic psychiatrist and on the theoretical and technical issues he believes analysts need to consider if they wish to be involved in social activism. There is considerable material included here that, to our knowledge, has not appeared in print before. While this printed interview provides invaluable insight, no single interview can fully capture the essence and greatness of Dr. Robert Jay Lifton. While Dr. Lifton was (to quote the title of his recent memoir) a "witness to an extreme century," we were witnesses to an extraordinary man who embraces extraordinary humanity.

Dr. Lifton has published numerous books and papers. Among those referred to in the course of the interview are the following: *Thought Reform and the Psychology of Totalism: A Study of "Brainwashing" in China* (New York: Norton, 1961); *Death in Life: Survivors of Hiroshima* (New York: Random House, 1968); *Home from the War: Neither Victims nor Executioners* (New York: Simon & Schuster, 1973); *Explorations in Psychohistory: The Wellfleet Papers* (edited with Eric Olson, New York: Simon & Schuster, 1975); *The Broken Connection: On Death and the Continuity of Life* (New York: Simon & Schuster, 1979); *The Nazi Doctors: Medical Killing and the Psychology of Genocide* (New York: Basic Books,

1986); *The Future of Immortality and Other Essays for a Nuclear Age* (New York: Basic Books, 1987); *The Protean Self: Human Resilience in an Age of Fragmentation* (New York: Basic Books, 1993); *Destroying the World to Save It: Aum Shinrikyo, Apocalyptic Violence and the New Global Terrorism* (New York: Holt, 1999); *Superpower Syndrome: America's Apocalyptic Confrontation With the World* (New York: Nation Books, 2003) and *Witness to an Extreme Century: A Memoir* (New York: Free Press, 2011).

JUDIE ALPERT: We are Judie Alpert and Elizabeth Goren, faculty members and supervisors of the NYU Postdoctoral Program in Psychotherapy and Psychoanalysis. We thank you, Dr. Lifton, for inviting us into your home to record this. Today we put ourselves in the shoes you have worn for nearly six decades. We interview you and you tell of being a psychiatrist and psychoanalytic researcher whose work made you, as you state in your most recent memoir, a witness to an extreme century.

ELIZABETH GOREN: You are a pioneer in bringing a psychoanalytically informed view to the public and to worldwide problems. We hope this interview will help our fellow professionals learn more about what psychoanalysis has to offer in dealing with world problems and with how individual psychoanalysts might find their own path to contributing to the public good.

JA: There are many analysts and others in the healing professions who have been inspired by you and your work.

EG: You have been what you called a "hidden," silent mentor to those of us who are trying to bring psychoanalytic thinking and sensibility to the world and to issues of contemporary society. That's why we wanted to interview you.

ROBERT JAY LIFTON: Well, in a way, from what you are both saying, I sense that you are responding to some effort on my part to bring professional work into passionate engagements with a society and against some of the dreadful things that were going on, especially the Vietnam War in the 1960s. And that has always been quite logical to me. But, you know, it has its difficulties and struggles. I have always tried to keep my passion, my social or political passion, connected to the professional effort and I have taken seriously the professional side, that of healing and understanding motivations, in relation to the activism. Psychoanalytic, psychological or psychiatric interviewers are partners in conversation and take on a special quality because it's where I live. I've tried to have my activism reach people in general but perhaps there is a special way in which it can reach colleagues.

JA: So, let's begin with psychoanalysis, since it's where you began your career. Please tell us about your education and training. But first, can you tell us whether you consider yourself a psychoanalyst?

RJL: No, technically, I'm not a psychoanalyst. I have to emphasize the paradox in my relation to psychoanalysis. Everything I've done in my research depends upon the existence of psychoanalysis. It would have been impossible without it, and yet at the time that I was beginning to do that work in the 1950s, psychoanalysis had already moved into a dominant but rigid position. On the one hand, I had all kinds of psychoanalytic influence from my reading, even before I went to medical school or entered psychiatry and psychoanalytic training. I've always lived with the idea that psychoanalysis is one of the great intellectual movements of the modern era, and the most advanced form of psychological training available. Yet I had a skeptical sense. It had a danger for me. If I didn't modify it and didn't feel free to move beyond its more rigid boundaries, it could undermine my perspective. And with my psychoanalytic training at the Boston Institute, again it was mixed. It did have a kind of closed atmosphere. Really pretty much only Freud was taught, as I remember it. There was something useful about confronting the prevailing orthodoxy of the time, in order to deepen one's own heresy.

By the time I went into psychoanalytic training, which was in the late 1950s, I think it was fortunate for me that I already had a beginning path, as I had done my first study of Chinese thought reform. The two and a half years or so in the institute in Boston were extremely valuable to me, but I didn't feel intellectually opened up by them. I felt supported by my analysis with respect to my struggles with family and other issues, but I didn't feel anything like a really lively intellectual atmosphere in that institute. Two and a half years later, after doing my Hiroshima study, becoming a psychoanalyst wasn't necessary for my kind of work. I still felt a certain amount of conflict with the psychoanalytic worldview as it was presented to me. Then I became part of a community of rather talented people who, like me, were deeply influenced by psychoanalysis, but freed in their way of looking at it, and not bound by psychoanalytic orthodoxy. A marvelous group of people—like Margaret Mead and Gregory Bateson, John Spiegel and Fritz Redl. Also David Riesman, who was one of my important mentors, and, of course, Erik Erikson. I became friendly with all of them. This sub-community of people valued psychoanalytic tradition powerfully but, at the same time, needed to be free of the orthodox demands.

My encounter with Erik Erikson went a long way toward, if not resolving it, kind of living with it and working from it. He was to me an exciting exemplar of a psychoanalyst, deeply steeped in psychoanalytic work, who could do this original work, and had this exciting perspective and could bring psychoanalysis into history. At the same time, we could talk about those rigidities in psychoanalytic orthodoxy and the spirit of openness, which in a way characterized some of the early movement. I felt that in my own struggles, and in Erikson's, that one's own work, one's own modified or heretical version of psychoanalytic work would be more superficial, less profound, if one didn't first encounter the power of what that movement had to convey, even in its rigidity.

EG: Relevant here is a question from one of the candidates in NYU's Postdoctoral Program in Psychoanalysis, Dr. Charles Arnheim. He asks about Erikson's influence on your work and why you think he is not more widely read at the present time.

RJL: Read Erikson if he attracts you. He'll come back. There are historical fads in psychoanalysis as in everything else and I think his work has sufficient power to reappear, and it's still around for a lot of groups. But I agree that it's sad in a way that he's not as vivid for many people now. That won't always be the case. With me, I experienced an "aha" moment or eureka experience in reading through his paper on ego identity while writing up my work on Chinese thought reform. In fact I'd read him before that. I had already read *Childhood and Society*, which had a lot of focus on identity. But what he so carefully and so brilliantly wrote in that paper spoke directly to my struggles to understand what I had encountered in the Chinese attempt to convert filial sons and daughters into filial Communists. He had a profound answer, of a kind I needed.

We are taught in psychoanalytic psychology or psychiatry that early childhood determines the rest of life and sometimes, when this is overdone, we get the sense that everything after the age of six or seven is mere superstructure. One of the many interesting things that Erik Erikson did in his portrayal of the life cycle is to give back a certain dignity to adulthood, in terms of change, learning and alteration, and a lot of my work has been focused on pressures in adulthood and the capacity for change and resilience in adulthood.

EG: It seems very clear that you took from psychoanalysis and went beyond it.

RJL: Well, what I found was that, despite all this contradiction and ambivalence, I learned a lot from psychoanalysis and developed my work from a modified psychoanalytic perspective. I found I could most deeply draw from the Freudian tradition by separating myself from the psychoanalytic institute. In my main theoretical book, *The Broken Connection*, I began to realize I was having a dialogue with Freud, in which I was struggling to find out more about death and its significance for psychology and psychiatry. Freud had a lot to say about that, but he said it in instinctual terms, and I was moving toward symbolizing terms. My point is that, in this struggle to learn more and find ways of moving ahead, I separated institutional psychoanalysis from intellectual psychoanalysis.

JA: But it informed your work, and your thinking.

RJL: It informed my work enormously, while requiring me to develop a different or modified psychoanalytically oriented perspective in my interview method and in general.

JA: What motivated you to do this work?

RJL: In one sense, I happened into it by being sent by the Air Force to Japan. I was drafted in the doctor draft and became a young, wet-behind-the-ears Air Force psychiatrist for a couple of years. My wife was in Japan with me and together we discovered the world. We started with Japan, but it was more than Japan. It was a culture outside the United States. It was just a different society, and when you are outside of your ordinary norm on an everyday basis you can often see the flux and the intensities in a society and the historical influences. So, I discovered the world through the military in that way, inadvertently.

Then with my last assignment, interviewing returning POWs (prisoners of war) when they were arriving in South Korea after being held by the Chinese, and on a ship taking them to San Francisco, one thing led to another. It was partly being thrust into the world, and partly seizing certain opportunities or moments. The motivations are complex. I became very interested in the thought reform process the POWs had been subjected to. I also had a sense of adventure. I wanted to do something interesting, and a little bit beyond the conventional, although I wasn't always courageous about plunging into it. The other thing that I'm realizing more and more, though I didn't write much about it in my memoir, is that this was a certain era in American history. There was the emergence in triumph from the World War II and an opportunity for adventurous Americans to experience the world.

In the early 1950s psychoanalysis connected with that triumphalism and became a power of its own in American society. Later I wrote critically about a lot of that, especially American hegemony or American triumphalism, or what I came to call the "superpower syndrome." But at that time, I was personally a part of it and benefited from it. That is, I became part of the occupation of Japan by being drafted. Like many other doctors and ordinary soldiers, I was sent to Japan and then into the Korean War. But I was well behind the lines, and had little to do with combat.

And so I was thrust into the world at a certain moment in American history, which was a big factor in what I did and became. It's true that lots of psychiatrists were sent by the Army or the Air Force to Japan and other places and didn't do these things. It was something that evolved in my developing identity as a psychiatrist out in the world, and that came in slow bits and pieces and then some plunges. Gradually, with lots of conflict, my identity as somebody who could do these things began to take hold. And that identity, that way of being, was very much influenced by my wife. We married rather young and she was there with me in all of these efforts. She buttressed and encouraged that identity, which would have been very hard, if not impossible, to evolve on my own.

JA: It sounds like she was very important to you and your work.

RJL: Very much so.

EG: How did your background and personal beliefs affect your choosing to work with the groups you worked with and how do you think your background impacted the people you worked with?

RJL: I came from a middle-class, Jewish background with a certain intellectuality, Rooseveltian liberalism and a third-generation immigrant sequence; my parents were American-born and trying to make their way in this society. Those things affected me in both my personal and evolving political and ethical life. Then in my own life, as well as my psychological probings, I began to try to find my place in connection with what I came to call an "allergy to totalism." There was something parallel between my political struggles and my psychoanalytic struggles, a sense of wanting to move ahead and break through as a critical voice, and to be critical of totalistic expressions of ideology. It's very important that it came at a certain moment in history.

You know, it's hard to analyze the significance of one's Jewish background and the kind of wandering openness you can sometimes find in Jewish intellectuals, but I wouldn't emphasize that so much. My focus has been on finding things that have universal significance. You always move to the universal by means of the immediate and specific. For instance, my Jewishness is very important to me, but I don't observe any religious principles and I would always want to see my Jewishness as my path to the universal, rather than my essence.

JA: Here's another big question: What do you really think about human nature?

RJL: I've studied some pretty ugly events. My friends, especially the skeptical, or let's say cynical ones, would corner me and say, "All right, Robert, now you've studied Nazi doctors, what do you think of human beings?" They wanted my answer to be "not very much." Instead I would say, I think we can go either way. That's always been my sense. I've studied horrendous forms of killing and violence and also impressive forms of resilience. I've met lots of people who have similar passions about justice and about confronting violence and killing. These acts of opposition are, I believe, expressions of hope. And so I've come to see us as human beings not wired to destroy ourselves in some absolute way, and not wired to live together in complete harmony in some absolute way, but wired for either possibility and for various combinations that we end up embracing.

JA: Would you say ordinary people are capable of atrocities?

RJL: We're all susceptible to group pressures and the potential for being socialized to group morés that are destructive. If you're a doctor or a psychiatrist in a hospital and the unit you are part of takes upon itself to do things that could be seen as destructive, such as treating people badly in the name of some principle, and you are part of that, you can be socialized to bad behavior. In the example I'm giving it may be very mildly bad behavior, but the same process can operate for more extreme forms of bad behavior. A major theme in my study of Nazi doctors was that journey from healers to killers, killing in the name of healing. I've been much concerned about professionals who can move toward destructive behavior as they adapt to environments in which this was the norm.

More recently, the example is all too vivid of American doctors and psychologists participating in torture, in Iraq and elsewhere. I knew that German doctors weren't unique in their vulnerability to being socialized to evil, but I didn't think, when I did that study, that I would later come upon American doctors who had been involved in torture. So, this capacity of ordinary people for being socialized to evil is strong and always needs our attention. I give a lot of focus to that capacity in us, in professionals, and perhaps in a special way, psychiatrists and psychologists who are supposed to be doing only healing work.

JA: What about Nazi doctors? They committed horrific atrocities. What would they say about it now, looking back on what they had done?

RJL: It was a little late when I initiated my study, which was in the late 1970s. A lot was known, but I extended that information by probing the psyches of some of these Nazi doctors. Fortunately, Alexander Mitscherlich, who had done an earlier exposé at the time of the Nuremberg trials in the 1940s, tutored me. He told me that the members of the Nazi generation, including the doctors, never could really take in psychologically what they had been part of, never could really confront fully what they had done, and therefore could almost never show genuine remorse. Instead, they called forth defense mechanisms of claiming that they were the victims or they were put in an impossible situation or that the Russians or somebody had victimized them. So I was kind of prepared because what I found when I visited most Nazi doctors was a man—those I interviewed were all men—who might have been mildly depressed and tried to present himself as not a Nazi, but a kind of burgher, a conservative citizen.

They hadn't been ideologues, most of them. With a few exceptions, like Mengele, who was a fanatic, most of them were ordinary and corruptible men. They had some elements of anti-Semitism; they had joined the Nazi party out of its promise of revitalization, i.e. becoming strong again both nationally and individually, and also out of ambition to make their way in the new movement, and then were corrupted in various ways. So, they were not extraordinary people. They were very ordinary.

I was surprised by how much they would talk. They talked a lot about what they did, what it was like if they were in Auschwitz, or if they were in a so-called "euthanasia" killing center, which was what I called direct medical killing. They could talk even rather openly, but they talked about it in a disassociated way as though the doctor himself and I were looking at a third person. It was a way of separating himself from that person who had been there some decades ago, in the camp or the "euthanasia" center or just practicing some form of Nazified medicine. It was a version of splitting, or what I called "doubling." None of them ever said to me, "What I did was evil, I feel terrible and guilty about it and feel great remorse about it." What a few could suggest instead, very indirectly, was something like this: "I'm glad that after the war I could deliver babies." They left out the rest of the sentence—bringing babies into life, rather than taking life away, as they had done.

The most culpable of them had been tried at Nuremberg or had died of old age. There were others who did things incrementally. I remember one doctor whom I interviewed who had at first protested against the experiments. When it was explained to him that the doctors needed to do this work on typhoid in order to prevent the German army from becoming ill and losing the war, he bought into that ideology and succumbed to the powerful group pressure. The fact that this is a possibility within the human repertoire makes the problem more demanding. It gives you an avenue for grasping how it happened. I say this as explanation, not as justification.

These were very ordinary people who incrementally moved toward doing what they did. That's what makes the Holocaust or any genocide a more difficult problem. When you recognize this capacity on the part of almost anyone to be socialized to evil, it is of great concern. We are not necessarily talking about radical anti-Semitism. Ordinary people can be socialized to do the things that the Nazis did. We must face this.

JA: Moving to a related area, how do communities heal and what can we do to aid the healing in individuals and communities?

RJL: The whole question of how communities heal, especially from atrocity, is a very big and difficult one and I don't have any magic bullet for that. I do know that healing from atrocity, from extreme trauma, requires coming to terms with some kind of meaning that one needs to give to that trauma. I have emphasized various aspects of the psychology of the survivor in my work, but particularly the need for a sense of meaning about that death encounter, or as I call it, that "death immersion." That's enormously important for the individual person who is always in some kind of community. Very often people so greatly traumatized, or who have survived death in a very searing manner, need one another because they sense a deep understanding or empathy for what they have been through. That's been true for Holocaust survivors, Vietnam War veterans, Hiroshima survivors, and, in fact, for all of the groups that I've studied.

Yet sometimes they can be uneasy about living in a community dominated by survivors, or people traumatized like they themselves are, and they need to move out of it. There can be painful struggles in all of that. With the case of Hiroshima, people would sometimes try to "pass," to cover over their exposure to the bomb, because they wanted to get away from it. There was also a pragmatic reason. They could be discriminated against for jobs and in other ways. It was thought that they were vulnerable to after-effects of radiation from the bomb. But even beyond that, there can be a desire to emerge from a psychological sense of taint that can be attributed to, or experienced by, survivors.

Perhaps any healing process seems to require a combination of confrontation and meaning-making in the death encounter, and at the same time moving beyond the death encounter into some dimension of renewal. It can be taking that meaning into a mission, such as when parents of children who die from leukemia dedicate their lives to contributing to leukemia research in some way. There can't be a more painful experience for parents. Survivors of Hiroshima can take on a mission of telling their story to the world as a warning. In this way the mission takes on a healing quality and functions as a service to others by conveying their knowledge, their special knowledge. Survivors of extreme trauma have to find their own way and they have to do it in some group process. It's often erratic and unpredictable and you can't fully direct it.

I was involved in this, in a very hands-on fashion, with Vietnam veterans. With other psychologists and psychiatrists and social workers, we came together with the vets and formed so-called rap groups, in which we talked a lot about the Vietnam War and about their lives in general. We learned a lot from them, and they presumably from us. We could see that process of healing taking shape in very moving ways right before our eyes and that was a real lesson in the healing of very traumatized people. It didn't always work perfectly and it could be erratic as I said, but it was moving nonetheless.

JA: Turning to your work on thought reform, which raises the question: can change be coerced?

RJL: I found in my studies that Chinese thought reform was never completely successful. It could set the boundaries for behavior in China. Perhaps a relatively small group was converted in a rather successful process, and another group at the other end resisted it and was troubled by it, and a larger in-between group was affected by it, but much less than totally converted. Exposure to thought reform taught people what they could do and not do in that society. And then, the Chinese did something strange, they over-reformed. They couldn't stop reforming because they were a religious-like movement, and if you are a religious-like movement, you often can't stop your evangelical impulses. They were like that with thought reform, and they often antagonized people in over-reforming.

At the time I did my original studies in the mid-1950s, thought reform was at its zenith. Since then the Chinese do much less of it. They still do it, and they still hold it in abeyance, as a kind of totalistic possibility. They do it to groups that they feel are threatening or to people considered deviants and it's seen as primarily punitive. It doesn't have that central position or that strong element of exhortation that they had in their more ideological phase. In fact, over that half-century, which is not a very long time historically, I've been amazed at watching China go from an ideologically centered state, seeking absolute purity of thought, into a commercially oriented society in which nobody believes the ideology anymore.

JA: Are there some people though who are more susceptible to thought reform?

RJL: Yes, I mean, people have very different needs. There are Westerners who have had a more brutal version of it in prisons with lots of physical brutality. There are many variables that can affect things. For example, if your whole sense of identity or sense of self is more uncertain or deeply confused, or if you have a tendency toward totalism, or the degree to which you've been brought up to examine ideas and look critically at things is limited, all these can affect susceptibility.

Also, it has to do with the intensity of the process to which you're subjected. One thing I've learned through all my research is an enormous respect for extreme environments. If the environment is powerful enough, individual differences become less important and people will react similarly to the environmental dictates. So, in my work, I focus less on individual idiosyncrasies than on the specifics of thought reform, of Hiroshima trauma, or of Auschwitz. I focus more on the nature of those extreme environments in relation to human beings, on the creation of these environments and on what they do to human beings. That has been my mission.

JA: Returning to the issue of totalism and dogma in psychoanalysis. Can you say more?

RJL: Yes, sure. First let me say that the word totalism, as used in psychological work, was Erikson's, and he meant all-or-none tendencies that could be observed in individual adolescent and young adult patients. Later he began to use it in some writing about Nazi Germany. But then I took it up and applied it, especially ideologically, and I called it "ideological totalism." There were the extreme examples of it in Chinese thought reform particularly, and that was not only totalistic but also even apocalyptic. They wanted to eliminate all language, all thought, that wasn't Communist or Maoist. You know, that's a wildly impossible goal, but that's what an apocalyptic goal can be.

I also became interested in much more limited forms of behavior that veered toward totalism, forms of re-education in which the environment is telling you that you are supposed to believe in a certain set of principles or rules. The re-education for that process involves patterns of criticism and self-criticism or even a kind of confession if you didn't think the right way. That kind of tendency was more common than the more extreme forms. For instance, it was picked up in regard to cultic movements in this country, but even in graduate programs, or in religious expressions, you could find elements of totalism, or elements of near-totalism where people avoided being buried in it by coming up for air.

I began to think about psychoanalytic training in this way, and I had a lot of conversations with Erikson, and by then there were a number of critiques by others of psychoanalytic training. I thought I could bring something to that critique. Rebel that I am, writing my first book was a way of bringing these issues together. I did it with considerable respect for psychoanalysis, talking about it as a great humanitarian movement of the modern era, which, in its origins, really focused on freeing the individual and encouraging the mind's capacity for openness and for new dimensions. But then, where one built institutional structures to further it, it could fall into some of the problems of other intense institutional structures that came from religion or other aspects of society. I focused on certain things, specifically the fact that upon entering a psychoanalytic institute, one was simultaneously patient, student and candidate. This meant that those in charge could make judgments that affected the core of one's psyche and extended into one's life indefinitely into the future, about whether one could pass muster and be accepted as a psychoanalyst. There was a danger that acceptable behavior, being approved as a psychoanalyst, depended upon the holding of correct beliefs, those of the ideological orthodoxy.

And I took up certain terms, like "resistance," "transference," "reality," and talked about how these could be manipulated by someone who thought that he or she possessed the truth in a belief system. There were and still are some psychoanalysts who believe that. These things are not so shocking as I say them now; maybe they weren't even then, because people were thinking those things. I felt that I had, in my research on thought reform, a model in its very extremity for lesser tendencies that had parallels to that model. In the end it wasn't all that shocking. Nobody wrote me angry letters or threatened me. My subsequent relationship with psychoanalysis as an institution has been one of live and let live, and I have frequently spoken at events sponsored by psychoanalytic institutes.

EG: I have a question related to what you've talked about here in terms of totalism and fundamentalism. How do you connect McCarthyism to what was happening in psychoanalysis then?

RJL: Well, psychoanalysis is so unusual and it's difficult to characterize politically. Certainly, every psychoanalyst I knew considered himself or herself an enemy of McCarthyism. I think McCarthyism violated the best spirit within psychoanalysis, which had to do with openness and freedom of thought. But psychoanalysis could veer toward McCarthyite totalism in certain institutional expressions or individual attitudes representing orthodoxy. There could be considerable nastiness toward people viewed as heretical. Otto Rank, Erich Fromm, Heinz Kohut and Carl Jung were some of those considered heretics. There were bitter sectarian battles within psychoanalysis and I think they had to do with totalizing one's own claim to truth.

Whether it comes from religion or intellectual life or some kind of healing procedure, what is common in totalism is a claim to absolute truth and an equal claim to absolute virtue. Those are dangerous claims. I think psychoanalysis has had the potential to extricate itself from that because it has a spirit of freedom, which Freud, at his best, represented.

JA: Moving to a different area, the intergenerational transmission of trauma and, specifically, transmission at the community level. Can you comment on that?

RJL: Yes, I think we've all learned to think more intergenerationally and perhaps in most of psychoanalytic work that's done within families. But as you're implying, it extends out into communities and into history. Once you think generationally, you're taking a step out further into history and that's what I try to do. It was certainly what Erikson tried to do before me, and what the group on psychology and history that Erikson and I formed together at Wellfleet, Massachusetts, way back in the mid-1960s did. It makes sense that subsequent generations will be influenced by trauma. It was very notable in Hiroshima, partly because it was physicalized in the danger of radiation effects, which can be transmitted across the generations. So there was real danger and much fear. For the most part, these effects have not materialized but it has been a terrible fear.

There has been more study of transgenerational issues in Holocaust survivors. Often the second generation of survivors of the Nazi death camps could never quite grasp what their parents had been through. They knew it was something dreadful. Their parents didn't really want to talk about it in many cases, partly because it was so painful and partly because they wanted to protect their children from this. The survivors wanted their children to be born free of it, but that could intensify the confusion and the anxiety on the part of the next generation, wondering about this horrible experience that had haunted their parents and needing to know something more about it. In these studies there has developed more recognition of the need for dialogue between the generations. Otherwise it's a suppressed history, and secrets over the generations can almost always be damaging.

Children of Nazis have been brought together with children of Holocaust survivors, and they've had fascinating encounters, finding they have much in common with each other. They couldn't be more different in what they came from, but in each case there's been an interruption of history, you might say, as transmitted over the generations. The parents of the children, parents who were Nazi functionaries, couldn't or wouldn't describe that in detail to their children.

I had one experience like this. I interviewed a middle-aged woman, who was the daughter of Eduard Wirths, who was the chief camp doctor at Auschwitz. She was in her forties, had two children and was rather sympathetic to me. She was willing to see me, all the more so because she had pain of her own, having to do with her learning gradually about information that had been kept from her for quite a while. She learned that her father had been the chief doctor at Auschwitz and that he had killed himself at the end of the war. She talked about sitting on the knee of her loving father in Auschwitz. Her father had been considered a good man, a kind and very conscientious doctor. He had embraced the Nazi movement and had been sent to Auschwitz, where, when he found the horrors there, reacted by improving the situation, improving the whole structure of medicine and medicalized killing. At the end of a really interesting interview she said, "Dr. Lifton, I want to ask you one question: 'Can a good man do bad things?'"

This is a very heavy and difficult generational transmission because there can be love between the generations even though the younger generation may have deep antipathy to, and even revulsion toward, what the older generation did. In her case, she and her brother were trying very hard to salvage something from that love to see what was real about that love, coming from a father who had done these dreadful things.

JA: You have said that survival "can close you down or open you out." Could you say more about that?

RJL: Yes, I've long been interested in the psychology of the survivor and I like the rhetoric of the survivor even more than simply trauma. Of course we need the rhetoric of trauma, too, but the survivor has that imagery and energy toward affirmation of life; staying alive is a powerful accomplishment in many such situations. With the survivors whom I have studied, beginning with my work on Hiroshima, I've come to a grid, or a set of psychological characteristics. One is the indelible image that a survivor retains and has to do with a death imprint. Another is a kind of self-condemnation, sometimes called survivor guilt or death guilt, a paradoxical form in which the person who has suffered or been treated brutally may feel guilty or at least may condemn himself or herself for staying alive while others died or for not having done more to help them. Another characteristic is the struggle with feeling, or what I call "psychic numbing" or diminished capacity or inclination to feel. Still another is a suspicion of counterfeit nurturing, a kind of hunger for help but resistance to being helped because it's equated with weakness. And the most important characteristic of the survivor is an overall need to find meaning in the death encounter in order to find meaning in life in general.

These elements can immobilize a survivor with an absence of meaning and an inability to pursue an affirmative, life-enhancing survivor mission. Meaning may come from love relationships or family or other connections beyond the self. All of that helps determine whether the survivor gets stuck in the death immersion, so to speak, and closes down. Or, whether the survivor confronts the death immersion, learns from that experience, takes hold of some special knowledge and opens out.

EG: Related to this issue of survival and the confrontation with death, we have a question from one of our former NYU graduate students, Andrea Rihm. She wrote: "Once you wrote that through your work you realized the symbolization of life and death is what we're all about. Nonetheless, nowadays the denial of death appears to be widespread. Do you think this might have any effect on the way we deal with trauma or social trauma?"

RJL: The denial of death is always widespread. Always has been. Always will be. America has its own set of institutions, or structured denial. Maybe more than other countries, but there's lots of denial of death everywhere and it does affect behavior. Just to take a very bold, simple example: consider the tyrants who seem to have this unspoken assumption that they'll live forever. Sometimes it's necessary to kill a lot of other people in order to reassert one's illusion of physical immortality. You can find all kinds of examples. Others have written about this.

But in my work about the symbolization of life and death, which you referred to in that question, there is this idea that we seek to see ourselves as part of something larger than the self. That's what I call "the symbolization of immortality." There's a real sense in which we feel ourselves to live on in our children and their children and in the communities that we become part of. We live on in our creative lives, through our influences on students and perhaps patients and on those who read our work or any kind of influence we may have upon other people in this life. Some of us can have a sense of living on through a religious principle and also through what all societies look upon as eternal nature, that we're part of nature. This is not to deny the fact of physical death, which we struggle to acknowledge and take in and accept. Our capacity to accept our own mortality is, in my view, enhanced by our ability to symbolize these larger forms of human connectedness. And that's where the symbolization of life and death becomes the central paradigm for my work.

EG: How has your work impacted you personally as well as professionally?

RJL: Of course it would be impossible not to have studies like these affect one, and they have. They've brought me, at moments, lots of pain and lots of sadness. They've also taken me into realms of absurdity, into gallows humor, and into the realms of poetry and literature. It's hard to summarize what they've done to me, but they're part of me and part of my life, and have acquainted me with forms of experience that have value. At first, I was kind of stunned when the people who had been through Hiroshima or Auschwitz, and one couldn't imagine worse experiences than those two, emphasized to me how much they valued the experience. It seemed like a strange word, you know, for what they had been through.

I've had no pain like that of survivors of Hiroshima or Auschwitz, but just by entering into their experiences, by being a witness to them, I've learned something of value, of profound value, about those experiences. In terms of my professional life, the work has taken me in a very idiosyncratic direction as a psychiatrist or psychological researcher, out there in the world, and that's had a lot of satisfaction for me. It's been a path that I've been fortunate to be able to follow. I've been helped by lots of marvelous friends and family, and especially my wife, in that process. Professionally I don't have regrets. I have had continuous satisfactions combined with struggles. Things don't stand still and the effort is never easy or without a certain amount of pain or conflict.

EG: What were the most momentous events you encountered and what were the most difficult testimonies that you've taken?

RJL: The work with Nazi doctors caused me the deepest pain by far, but an equally momentous event for me was my exposure to survivors in Hiroshima much earlier. The exposure in Hiroshima was in 1962, and the Nazi doctors in 1978, 1979. The Hiroshima immersion changed my life. It created a kind of prism or lens through which I see the world as being threatened by ultimate weaponry all the time. I've experienced lifelong passion and responsibility to confront that threat in extending my work from the Hiroshima study.

My work on Nazi doctors was just very painful to see through, to go through these interviews. Of course it has stayed with me and had particular intensity for me as a Jew, though one didn't have to be a Jew to do that work or feel that intensity. The experience took me deepest into direct, hands-on evil. It's not always clear what one learns from evil, but one learns something important.

People, including psychoanalysts, often like to stay away from these issues. I can understand that feeling, but I believe strongly in confronting them. There's a sense in which, even if you try to stay away from them, they're still there. If you confront them, there's a slight freeing of the self, or maybe more than slight because one is no longer as burdened by the denial of how our world has functioned. That's at least the approach I have.

EG: So it's been, in a certain way, liberating for you.

RJL: Yes, there have been elements of that but it wouldn't be liberating if I just did it by myself and was alone in being immersed in these things. Having friends who understood these things has been important to me.

Even more so, a wife who was a life partner for so long. We did much together and yet had separate careers. All this brought a certain quality of experience that wouldn't otherwise have been there. One can call it liberating, one can derive satisfaction from probing areas that are hard to deal with and that others resist, from having gone out into the world and lived out certain struggles and adventures.

EG: You're saying that part of what was helpful was being with other people. This was just what you were talking about earlier about the survivors healing in groups, in connection.

RJL: Yes, and we all form groups in order to experience our intellectual and professional life, as well as our personal life, our family and our friends. My work has been an avenue to groups I've helped create, which included people with extraordinary qualities, people with unusual concerns of this kind. I've worked in an academic setting but when we form what can be called "deep colleagueship," it's rarely done through ordinary everyday function. The deep colleagueship is experienced when you are confronted together with a strongly ethical issue, often a political one—like, say, psychologists and psychiatrists and torture, or something like that, and working together on it. We have a sense of joining in with each other, group function at its best, that's special and that doesn't occur in the everyday arranging of courses or details that we might otherwise carry out. So, I've had certain intellectual groups and friendships that have been inseparable from the kind of work I've done, that have really meant a lot to me.

EG: Can you say a little more about how your work has affected your personal confrontation with death and sense of mortality?

RJL: Yes, the work has been much concerned with death and with struggles to affirm life in the face of death. It doesn't mean that I'll display some unusual or profound courage in the face of death, but it does mean that I can be a little bit informed by what I've learned and that has value.

EG: We've been focusing on how your research has challenged and transformed you. I'm wondering about all the people you've interviewed. Do you think the interview process was therapeutic in some way for them?

RJL: All of the interviews I've done, which have been research interviews with strong elements of dialogue, have had give-and-take in them and therapeutic components. I've worked a lot with people who have been traumatized or exposed to extremely painful situations related to death, or threatened death, and so they responded, for the most part, to a therapeutic perspective. But, for such a therapeutic perspective, and with research of the kind that I've tried to do, it's also very important to immerse oneself in the subject one is studying. I couldn't bring a psychoanalytic perspective to Chinese thought reform without immersing myself in that process and for that matter, in twentieth-century and earlier Chinese history as well. Similarly I couldn't have had anything like a therapeutic effect on the Hiroshima survivors unless I knew something about Japan, about those atomic bombings, and unless I could share with them a beginning understanding of the effects on people.

We're not here, as psychological professionals, just to enlighten people. We learn our psychological perspective and have to add to that specific knowledge about what we are taking on and share it with people. I've learned a tremendous amount about each issue I've studied from the people who've been through it. They have been my teachers in terms of the experiences they've had.

EG: Let's talk about your future work.

RJL: I hope to think through more and do more research on how war begets war and how that vicious circle of war-making can be interrupted. It doesn't mean that anything I write will suddenly cancel out wars. It means that it could contribute, limitedly, to certain forms of knowledge about what we do and perhaps about how we can contest warlike meanings. So, it would again be more intellectual work or scholarship and some element of activism, I think.

EG: Would it involve interviewing?

RJL: Well, I'm not sure now whether I want to do any interviewing. I've done most of my major studies through interviews, but I have done other studies without interviews in more theoretical ways, and I have to think through what seems right for me at this point. I could imagine doing it either way. But if I don't interview people, I could still take various materials from moments of history. Perhaps again focusing on the Vietnam War, which I believe still haunts our society, and affects all of our war-making and perhaps much of our resistance to war-making.

EG: How do you envision our future world? And how do you think that developing technology is going to impact future violence?

RJL: Well, I don't have any grand statements to make about that, but I have been preoccupied with the technology of killing. That means hydrogen bombs, and that is such a quantum leap in the technology of murder. It affects everything in our time. So, one thing I've been doing recently is conducting a dialogue, a kind of debate with people, notably Steven Pinker, who emphasize an increasingly peaceable world and speak of the improving situation in relation to diminishing numbers of wars and diminishing violence. In contrast, I see our technological revolution as so dangerous that these earlier statistics have dubious relevance for it. I've written and spoken a little bit about it and will continue to work on these issues.

I'm also concerned with immediate American behavior in Afghanistan and the recent atrocities of Sgt. Bales and others, which reflect what I call an "atrocity-producing situation." I hope to write something about that in connection with our whole relation to the Afghanistan War, really the American way of war, from Vietnam to Iraq to Afghanistan, even though they are different wars. And then I hope to do some more work on the subject of how war begets war, specifically focusing on what determines the direction of meaning structure, that is, toward or away from further war-making. The meaning structures formed by survivors in their death encounter can vary.

For instance, when My Lai, a big atrocity in the Vietnam War, was revealed to the American people in 1969, there were two groups of Holocaust survivors who were on the public stage. One of them was a group of Auschwitz survivors, who, rather humbly and movingly, sought to find a way to make a statement of protest about My Lai because, as different as it was from Auschwitz, it was coming too close. On the other hand there was a group of quasi-fascist Holocaust survivors headed by a man named Meir Kahane, who, under the slogan, "Never Again," took it upon themselves to have the right to be violent toward Arabs or Palestinians who disagreed with them and to consider them "Nazis." So, this was the same event, the Holocaust, with a completely different survivor meaning. You could say the same of Vietnam, from which most of us took a survivor meaning, even when we were survivors from a distance: don't ever get into wars like that. But others, who named themselves the Vulcans, and were advisors to George W. Bush, took the opposite meaning: you must express more power; you must project more strongly American military power on the world. One could see the Iraq War and, to some extent the Afghan War, as related to survivor meanings and survivor missions from Vietnam.

So, I'm interested in how alternative views to war-making and preventing war-making can take hold. Although there has always been this traditional warrior ethos or survivor meaning from war—you must get back at the enemy and do the unfinished work of those killed, by fighting the next war—I'm encouraged by the fact that there have also always been opposite survivor meanings of the warrior hero. That opposite meaning involves protesting the war and saying, "It's not worth it." Even in the *Iliad*, there were plaintive cries, not only on the part of women but also from Achilles himself, the warrior hero, protesting the war and saying, in effect, "It's not worth it." That's the alternative survivor mission from war-making, and of course it's the one that I've tried, and will continue to try, to contribute to.

EG: And do you see that as intergenerationally transmitted?

RJL: Well, there's no doubt that it is intergenerationally transmitted because fathers of the Vietnam veterans were veterans of World War II. They bounced their sons on their knee and told them about their glorious achievements in World War II. And of course it was a war where there was a real evil out there that America felt it had to fight. So the son would sit on his father's knee and wait for his moment to come, where he could demonstrate his male courage.

Vietnam veterans did something quite extraordinary; they turned against their own war and developed a survivor meaning to the effect that the war was meaningless, that it had no justification; in that sense they were trying to interrupt the warrior ethos. And to some limited extent they have. The anti-war Vietnam veterans have tutored some of the Iraq veterans, who are the next generation of warriors. Some have worked with, and learned from, the Vietnam veterans and have formed anti-war groups. So, these issues are transmitted intergenerationally, but the interruption of the warrior ethos by the Vietnam veterans was partial and overcome and contested by other expressions of the warrior ethos. You never solve it once and for all or have that moment when everything is in place beautifully. It's a process and a continuing struggle.

EG: Do you think it could be overcome?

RJL: I think it could be partially overcome. And that is an expression of hope.

Note

1 Reprinted from *Psychoanalysis, Culture & Society, suppl. Special Issue: Psychoanalysis, Trauma, and Community* 18.2 (Jun 2013): 199–216 by permission of Palgrave Macmillan.

Chapter 10

My Fulbright journey

Mary-Joan Gerson

My journey to Namibia in the summer of 2012 was as a "Fulbright Specialist." Since the award did not have a "psychologist" category, I applied under the "public health" designation. I believe that my credentials as a psychoanalyst and family therapist, my articles and presentations on chronic medical illness as well as working with physicians in collaborative health care models, made me attractive as a third world health consultant (Gerson, 2009). I was asked to teach in the Psychology Department of the University of Namibia as well as at the medical school (of the University of Namibia), both located in the capital city, Windhoek. But I extended my work at the University by consulting at a psychiatric and a general medical hospital and I met with a group of social workers in the Namibian Department of Health. Additionally, during my month's stay I met with various non-governmental organization (NGO) representatives and mental health care professionals.

My husband and I had been in the Peace Corps in Nigeria in the late 1960s and we very much wanted to return to West Africa. He is a physician and became a Fulbright Specialist as well, and thus we were able to process this experience together. Though we waited patiently, no opportunity materialized in West Africa, and the Fulbright office asked us—about two months before we hoped to leave—if we were interested in going to Namibia. It was an unknown country to me. I was shocked to learn one week before departure that Namibia had suffered a full-blown apartheid regime, functioning virtually as a protectorate of South Africa until it became independent as late as 1989.

What was most significant for me in my one-month immersion as a Fulbright Specialist, specifically from a psychoanalytic perspective? First, the gap between what my expectation of what my second African immersion

would be and the reality of my Namibian experience; second, how crucial it was to privilege inquiry over acquired expertise when entering a new culture; and third, the challenge of moving forward toward making a meaningful contribution while tolerating considerable ambiguity and uncertainty.

Windhoek, itself, was something of a shock for me. My internal representation of an African city was imprinted by my prior Peace Corps experience in Nigeria (from 1965–1967) where I worked in a child mental health clinic and did research for the World Health Organization. I did spend my first year in Nigeria in the capital city, Lagos. However, Lagos and Windhoek are intergalactically different. What was so startling about Windhoek? The morning after I arrived I had an appointment with a psychologist at the University who herself had been awarded a US government Fulbright award to study at Howard University. I pictured us meeting in a version of downtown Lagos, Nigeria—music blaring from every storefront, the streets crowded with shoppers in vibrant varieties of patterned headdresses and tunics. Instead I found myself drinking cappuccino in an elegant café, surrounded by tables of cheerful, animated groups of colleagues and friends, but these tables were largely segregated by race. The difference between these two urban contexts and the national histories they represented became a conundrum that I dealt with throughout my month's immersion in Namibian culture. How familiar to us as psychoanalysts is the struggle between the internally coded, and the jarring reality of external experience. In fact I think the tension between the resolutely expected and the startling freshness of new experience lies at the heart of psychoanalytic work. The discrepancy makes our work difficult and sometimes painful, but its resolution is personally strengthening. I never really knew how much my preoccupation with apartheid and race in Namibia emerged from the contrast to my Nigerian Peace Corps experience, since Namibians, as I will discuss, were not very eager to make either subject a focus of public, nor even private, discussion. I was never really sure how much I glossed my Namibian experience with my own sense of personal uneasiness. However, this is an inevitable and constant dilemma we struggle with psychoanalytically.

Dr. Mara Mberira, my university host, did broach the legacy of apartheid that first morning. She talked about generations of inadequately educated professionals that necessitated importing professionals from other African countries. Though very much needed at a certain point in Namibian history, the (former) African expatriates were no longer willing to transfer power to Namibian Ph.Ds and M.Ds. I was shocked to learn that there was only one white student registered at the University of Namibia—a very bright psychology major I'm happy to report. Where do the others go to study? To the universities in Cape Town, South Africa, although the University of Namibia is actually a fine academic institution.

Dr. Mberira and I had already engaged in Skype conversations about lectures and consultations I might offer. Once again in our first breakfast meeting, she described prevalent and, to my ears, immense psycho-social problems: violence against women, drug abuse, and a high HIV prevalence. I left our meeting not only preoccupied with apartheid but deeply humbled by the gap between my own clinical knowledge and the magnitude of the social problems I would be addressing in my classes and consultations. However, my anxiety about being a good enough fit for this academic responsibility had already been tempered by a crucial consultation.

I had been urgently collecting teaching materials and tapes on domestic violence (not a specialty of mine), HIV counseling (not a specialty of mine), and addiction (equally not) in the two weeks before my departure when I learned that a mentor of mine, Salvador Minuchin, was in New York and available for a visit. His advice was particularly useful. He asked, "Why don't you teach what you know best, show the tapes you favor, and ask the students how your thoughts and clinical perspective apply to Namibian culture?" My roots in interpersonal psychoanalysis have always favored inquiry (Levenson, 1988), a dedicated probing at what lies beyond the security buffer of a too comfortably personified sense of self and relationship. Thus shifting my expertise to inquiry from mastery felt familiar and organic.

I had described my principal interests to Dr. Mberira, including psychodynamic therapy, family therapy, attachment theory, and coping with chronic illness, and I found a full schedule of lectures waiting for me when I arrived. I taught these subjects to undergraduate psychology and undergraduate social work students. These are the students who become the primary counselors dealing with all the significant Namibian social issues; the psychology major requires two years of specialization, and health psychology, three. I was consistently impressed with the level of discussion of my classes. I was particularly struck by their quick assimilation of family systemic concepts, and I wondered whether a culture of extended family structure and tribal complexity fosters systemic reflection. Only once was I greeted with a hostile reception. Early on, a student clearly supported by a coterie of her friends, asked if I were surprised that they actually used computers in

Namibia, and another wondered "why I came." I learned that the United States had a checkered profile in Namibia. We are an attractive democracy but we followed a political course of support for South African oppression.

Naturally when my students and I talked about family dynamics, we entered into discussion of some of Namibia's most pressing social issues, for example the one-parent, female-headed home. I tried to discuss the reason for father abandonment, which I saw very much related to demoralization in male identity during the apartheid era. It was men who went to the cities to work, living in tribally segregated townships, generally alone. What more sinister way to destroy a sense of family cohesion? We talked about the prevalence of domestic violence in Namibia. In fact, I visited the National Legal Center, an NGO with primarily British support, and read through a recent report on domestic violence. I learned that in a recent survey, one-third of young Namibian men had endorsed physical punishment for a wife who refuses sex, burns food, or fails to manage children competently. The phenomenon of domestic violence is a very dense one in terms of cultural history, since it seems that the tribal traditions of the eight countries in Southern Africa characteristically sanctioned physical aggression against wives. In these discussions, I had to effortfully keep my mind open and my thinking fluid, determined to privilege the space for exploration that the students and I were entering together. I had to keep in check my own assumption that domestic violence had been sustained and perhaps intensified due to the demoralization of husbands and the ongoing alarming rate of male unemployment, which reaches up to 40 percent of the adult population. What was striking to me was the reluctance of the students to talk about the potentially demoralizing effects of apartheid, and the indication that their parents avoided this discourse as well. Namibians read the recent history of South Africa and Zimbabwe as a cautionary narrative, and they are committed to avoiding the chaos and disruptions of these neighboring countries. A common assumption is that keeping discussion of possible apartheid sequelae under the carpet will be beneficial to national cohesion. As a psychologist I question this, since I believe that modulated, carefully shaped discussions of traumatic experience can result in collective understanding and potential healing. But I recognized that I was carrying a psychoanalytic presumption about the intergenerational transmission of trauma (Bradfield, 2011). I reassured myself that as long as I kept in view the frame I had imported to Southwest Africa, and not assumed that it was imprinted in the Namibian collective psyche, I would stay honest and flexible. Isn't this what our clinical work always demands?

Of course we covered more ordinary dynamic conundrums, though in these discussions I had to keep a keen ear open to new and culturally specific contexts. Students frequently talked about the complexity of being raised, often for a significant part of their childhood, in the homes of other members of their extended family and how different expectations and disciplinary styles can be confusing and conflictual. There were other class discussions that were suddenly almost shockingly familiar, for example, the difficulty of having men express their feelings in psychotherapy. I sometimes felt I ricocheted between the universal and the local in a kind of pell-mell fashion.

Another focus of my Specialist consultation was with social workers from the Ministry of Health, with whom I met on several occasions. I spent a day at the local city hospital of Windhoek, making rounds and observing interviews of the social work staff, but my most useful engagement were group conversations that focused on health psychology issues. Namibia has a very high AIDS prevalence, perhaps 20 percent of the population, higher than South Africa's at this point. Medication and counseling are free, but these interventions are subverted by the evangelical ministers and native healers of Namibia who frequently do not believe in the medical approach to AIDS. When patients return to their villages they are counseled to throw away medication and resume herbal and spiritual treatment, or devote themselves to prayer. The social workers and physicians involved in treatment are profoundly discouraged. Here again, I had to counter my own angry frustration at this treatment disjuncture. I couldn't altogether desist from thinking about a solution since, after all, this was a socio-political dilemma, not a psychoanalytic engagement.

I raised the possibility of a conference engaging native and religious leaders along with Western-trained physicians and counselors to find a way to respect different expertise and to collaborate rather than battle each other. I was told that a conference of this kind had been held years before, that the translation across the three predominant tribal languages was arduous and had accomplished little. In other conversations with this group we talked about rituals of grieving across tribal traditions. In this particular meeting, I realized that I offered the advantage of being an outsider: I could open up the issue of tribal differences, historical rivalries, and current tensions, because I was unaffiliated. Tribal tensions is a topic avoided in professional, collective discussions, but as opposed to apartheid, is quite accessible in private conversations.

Given space limitation I will not be able to describe some of the other connections I made: a visit to a local Peace Center, meeting with a young psychologist determined to invigorate the local psychological association, visits with two Peace Corps volunteers, one of whom worked in a disability program and the other in a daycare program for children, and a meeting in the north with a former South African family therapist who was planning to establish a family therapy treatment center in the heart of Namibia.

What was fascinating and unnerving to me as the month progressed was my own sense of how little I was able to really grasp and map the psychosocial reality of Namibian life. In this regard, Fulbright offered me a booster shot in tolerating uncertainty and experiencing humility. My working template was always on the verge of erasure and fracturing. For example, early in my stay I decided that the economic culture of Namibia was bimodal, an elite of affluent white citizens, top government employees, and corporate executives, juxtaposed to an underclass which was impoverished and unemployed. About three weeks into my stay, I had to purchase something and went to a shopping mall. It was filled with middle-class Black African families pushing heaping shopping carts. Certainly time for a revision, but what else was unknown or mistaken in my reading of this culture?

I was rerouted and redirected much of the time I taught and talked in Namibia but I rarely felt destabilized. My psychoanalytic training in self-reflection, privileging exploration, and tolerating uncertainty stood me well. The Fulbright Specialist experience was an incredibly invigorating experience and, above all, made me value my clinical identity and way of thinking in a way that I often take for granted in my busy, albeit richly textured, New York professional life

References

Bradfield, B. (2011). The dissociation of lived experience: a relational psychoanalytic analysis of the intergenerational transmission of trauma. *International Journal of Psychoanalytic Self Psychology*, 6, pp. 531–550.

Gerson, M.J. (2009). *The Embedded Self: An integrated psychodynamic and systemic perspective on couples and family therapy.* New York: Routledge (The Analytic Press), 2nd edition.

Levenson, E.A. (1988). The pursuit of the particular. *Contemporary Pyschoanalysis*, 24, pp. 1–16.

Chapter 11

Social trauma, politics and psychoanalysis

A personal narrative[1]

Nancy Caro Hollander

This chapter suggests that politics can be a portal to the world of psychoanalysis and that psychoanalysis can provide a lens through which to view the centrality of politics in psychological life. It is an essay about the personal and collective meanings of shared trauma and the journey toward resilience and reparation of political destructiveness. I explore these themes in an autobiographical essay that traces my evolution as a Latin American historian and feminist and Marxist activist whose professional and political experiences in the tumultuous conditions of revolution and dictatorship in Latin America inexorably led me to psychoanalysis. The particular psychoanalytic paradigm I had the good fortune to encounter in Latin America was a theory and praxis that was fashioned within extreme social situations of political repression and resistance, of human destructiveness and resilience. Its interest in the intersection between psychic and social reality represented continuity with the radical spirit of European psychoanalysis whose early roots were linked to bohemian, artistic and philosophical critiques of repressive bourgeois culture and to leftist political analyses of oppressive class-based sources of psychological misery (Jacoby, 1983; Damousi and Plotkin, 2012). This Latin American psychoanalysis I came to know represented theoretical principles and clinical innovations publicly identified with struggles for human rights and social justice. It has been a guiding force in the development of my life as a psychoanalyst, in which I have striven to integrate a radical political critique of social power and ideology with a psychoanalytic understanding of individual and group unconscious fantasy, affects and defenses.

A recent experience can set the scene for my exploration of this history. It is October 16, 2011, and I am back once more in Buenos Aires, which feels like home to me because of the central role it has played since the late 1960s in my personal, professional and political life. It is a balmy spring evening, and a group of psychoanalysts I have known for years has gathered in a colleague's home to share a meal and enthusiastic discussion about the psychosocial meanings of the uprisings of the millions of people, from Tunisia to New York, who are protesting the disastrous impact on their lives of corporate globalization. These Argentine psychoanalysts have a long history of progressive political activism that has taken them out of their consultation rooms to offer their psychological services to diverse populations in nontraditional settings and circumstances. They are eager to hear my report from the United States (US) because I have just arrived from participating in the inaugural Washington DC Occupy events. My videos vividly depict the excitement of the thousands who arrived in the US capital from everywhere in the country to take part in the innovative democratic general assemblies and colorful demonstrations that protest the many manifestations of the unjust and inequitable structures of US capitalism (Blumenkranz et al., 2011; Gitlin, 2012). My Argentine colleagues are intrigued and express their relief at witnessing evidence of consciousness among the popular classes in this country about the nature of the systemic sources of the escalating immiseration throughout the world, whose impact now extends to citizens within the heart of Empire itself. I am excited, after years of having lived with my Argentine colleagues through their country's tumultuous history, to demonstrate that more people in the US are understanding, and protesting against, some of the same exploitative political and economic forces that Latin Americans have militantly struggled against for decades. And I am glad to convey to my Argentine friends, in response to their queries, that a network of psychoanalysts within this country identifies with the concerns of the Occupy movement and are increasingly effective in creating a presence within the profession for a dialogue about the relationship between social and psychological pathology, intrapsychic and class conflict and models for reparative action (Layton, Hollander and Gutwill, 2006; Harris and Botticelli, 2010).

History, trauma and politics

As I recall the journey that led me to this October 2011 encounter, I keep in mind the effect of the present on the past and the paradoxical and nonlinear attributes of memory. My attempt to create a meaningful narrative that traces the evolution of my encounter with social trauma, from the pre-psychoanalytic period of my life to my psychoanalytically informed experience, must perforce contain elements of what Laplanche calls "afterwardsness." His elaboration of Freud's notion of *nachträglichkeit* and his discussion of history, time and memory show how we do not exist in one time frame, but rather simultaneously within an enigmatic tapestry of past, present and anticipated future all at once (Laplanche, 1999a, 1999b). The specific evidence for me of afterwardsness emerges whenever I write about my experiences in Latin America, during the course of which I oscillate between dissociative states to a familiar and repetitive sense of being haunted by traumatic losses whose mourning still feels incomplete and whose impact continues to guide my apprehensive concerns about today's traumatogenic social environment. So it is as I write this narrative about the beginnings of my journey some four decades earlier, when in October 1969 I arrived in Buenos Aires, a doctoral candidate in Latin American history, armed with a Fulbright dissertation fellowship and four years of experience in university activism in the anti-war, civil rights and women's liberation movements. In that era of rebellion all over the world, Argentina was fertile ground for my continuing intellectual and political development. For the next five years, I spent much of my time there, living through a series of military dictatorships, successful popular struggles that won a period of democratic governance and then the descent into the political and economic chaos that would produce a military coup and the state's infamous Dirty War against its own citizens.

As a graduate student I had studied the political economy of underdevelopment and the centuries-long history of reformist and revolutionary movements intent on altering the inequitable institutions responsible for the impoverishment and political impotence of the majority of the continent's peoples. Through my research travels in Latin America I had learned about the varied ways human beings respond to oppressive life circumstances. Through the lens of Marxist theory and the political philosopher Antonio Gramsci's work on hegemony, I observed in present tense what I had studied about the history of the continent: human beings' tendency, rooted in an identification with the dominant ideology and structures of power, to suffer from a passive acceptance of oppression. Yet this quiescence was punctuated at historical moments by a resilient capacity to develop critical consciousness and the courage to challenge authority (Boggs, 1984). My doctoral research focused on a specific aspect of these themes in the context of the gendered and class exploitation of women in Argentine dependent capitalism and their political mobilization during the twentieth century by socialist and feminist organizations as well as the Peronist women's movement.

When I arrived in Argentina, the country was under military rule (although moderate compared to the state terrorist regime that would govern after 1976). Often my research and access to relevant official resources were hampered, a limitation compensated for by the contacts I made with prominent intellectuals, scholars and political activists whose expertise and personal testimonies brought an exciting immediacy to my archival investigations. The military's erratic attempts at censorship failed to dampen Buenos Aires's rich intellectual life. The capital retained its customary role as a cultural mecca in which the latest trends in European culture provided a rich cross-fertilization in philosophy, arts, literature and cinema. Although I was not directly involved with the psychoanalytic community of Buenos Aires and did not know that it represented the fourth largest in the world, I could not help but be impacted by the centrality of psychoanalysis in the city's intellectual life. In this sophisticated Third World social environment, the Marx–Freud dialogue attracted intellectuals from many different fields and inspired fascinating conversations in popular culture as well as the academy (Hollander, 1990).

In this milieu I became familiar with what it feels like to live a quotidian existence that seems quite normative—one goes to work, takes care of children, socializes with friends and partakes in a variety of cultural activities—and at the same time experiences the threat produced by erratic evidence of a repressive state that enacts violence on any of its own citizens it views as a threat to the political status quo. By the early 1970s, my academic and political interests put me in touch with grassroots trade-union activists, political militants of small leftist parties and social radicals among professionals and artists, some of whom were working in community projects among the Argentine poor and the Bolivian immigrants inhabiting the appallingly impoverished "*villas miserias*" on the outskirts of Buenos Aires. Along the way I met Gabriella Christeller, an Italian feminist living in Buenos Aires, whose son was a leftist activist being held with many of his comrades as a political prisoner in the infamous Rawson Penitentiary located in Trelew in the distant south of Argentina. Gabriella and I established a women's organization called the Argentine Feminist Union. (The group's initials, UFA in Spanish, were the same as the Argentine expression meaning, "Enough, I've had it up to here.") The Buenos Aires literati and leftist intellectuals and activists, recently aware of the women's liberation movement in the US and Europe, flocked to the events we hosted and eagerly signed up for the consciousness-raising groups I facilitated.

Meanwhile, the political opposition to Argentina's military government, its status as a dependent capitalist country and the role of the US hegemon in its internal affairs, was becoming more widespread and organized. As legitimate possibilities for dissent were suppressed, increasing numbers of Argentines became completely alienated from the system and pushed for more radical strategies for change. Several armed revolutionary groups arose (mirroring developments throughout Latin America), with the goal of reviving political democracy and long-overdue economic reforms. Dissident voices within the Catholic Church coalesced in the Liberation Theology movement in which priests and nuns allied themselves with progressive political struggles. One such grouping, known as Third World Priests, organized national week-long encounters that brought together young male and female peasants and rural workers to educate them about their rights and the principles of organizing to achieve improvements in their dismal living and working conditions. I was invited to several of these *encuentros* to give workshops to help these young people become aware of the negative impact of gendered power dynamics on their identity and relationships and the consequent conflict and disharmony that weakened their ability to effectively reach their shared goals. I was deeply moved by the humanity of the religious activists who were training these young people from humble origins to become articulate leaders of local struggles for social justice in their rural communities throughout the country.

Increasing confrontations between these opposition forces and the state meant that we often went to sleep at night with the ominous sounds of exploding bombs and machine-gun fire piercing the silence. I was also now on occasion meeting individuals who had been arrested and tortured by the military or police. It was chilling to be in their presence, especially among those whose spirits had been broken irrevocably by the experience. Only later would I realize that one purpose of their imprisonment, torture and release was their function as a chilling reminder to those who came in contact with them of what awaited anyone who dared to challenge the authorities. In retrospect, I recognize that at the time I was able to manage the fear produced by such encounters because I was armed, one might say armored, by my political critique and commitment to social justice that included close bonds with others whom I admired and with whom I deeply identified. It seems to me now that I was able to function in this culture of fear and to ward off anxiety about personal risk and continue my activism because of the gratification of realizing an ego ideal by then deeply saturated by the era's revolutionary political ideals.

A particularly traumatic event illustrates this period's charged atmosphere. One evening in August 1972, Gabriella and I were about to host an encounter of the various small feminist groups that had emerged in Buenos Aires, when we received word that there had been an attempted prison break at Rawson Penitentiary and that, after giving themselves up, 16 prisoners had been shot down in cold blood by the marines. The names of the few who had successfully escaped as well as those who had been executed were not being released, nor were the victims' families being allowed to travel to the prison. Completely distraught because we knew nothing of the fate of Gabriella's son, we began the meeting with a proposal that all the groups join in a public denunciation of the government's actions and a demand that the families have access to information about their loved ones and contact with the several survivors of the massacre. I was shocked by the refusal of some of the women to criticize the military government on the grounds that they were opposed to all men, revolutionaries as well as dictators. Women, they insisted, were oppressed by virtue of their gender no matter what the political ideology of the men in their lives. I, like the majority of others present, held feminist views that included a Marxist perspective of the exploitative class relations that had produced the repressive military government, so that in spite of this minority sentiment, we decided to join the many organizations in the country protesting the state's actions. As it turned out, Gabriella's son was one of the fortunate survivors of the massacre. Several years later, I met another survivor of the Trelew Massacre, Maria Antonia Berger, a courageous woman whose face and body had been disfigured by the barrage of bullets that had almost killed her. I was in Buenos Aires in my role as a member of a Los Angeles-based film collective called Lucha Films, and I was filming Maria Antonia for a feature documentary we were making called *Communiqué from Argentina* (Bray, 2012). I never saw Maria Antonia again; some months after the military coup in 1976, along with thousands of other Argentines, she was disappeared and assassinated.

But between the Trelew Massacre and the Dirty War that would assault the body politic some four years later, a parenthesis occurred during which a hard-won return to democratic rule permitted the flowering of an openly radical cultural and political environment that made Argentina a compelling place to be. In neighboring Chile, the democratic socialist Allende government had also produced a cultural renaissance in which artists, poets, writers and musicians painted, wrote and sang in support of its reformist and anti-imperialist policies. But unfortunately this exhilarating political environment lasted a very brief period of time. By September 1973, in the wake of the horrendous military coup that overthrew Allende, I was interviewing refugees from Chile who were fleeing across the Andes to seek asylum in what was, for the moment, still a democratic Argentina. I felt it was my responsibility to translate and publish these interviews so that North Americans would know the truth of the central role our government was playing in the terrible repression overtaking Chile, and I pushed away feelings of dread as I listened to my interviewees' terrifying experiences. I spent several days with the writer Ariel Dorfman just after his escape from Chile. His manic state of mind, born out of what he had experienced in the early days following the coup, was contagiously destabilizing. Only later would I come to understand the mechanism of disavowal that I employed in order not to have to experience in myself the psychological implosion to which I might otherwise have submitted.

Indeed, as I traveled back and forth between Argentina and the US during that period, I believed I had an ethical obligation to raise consciousness in this country about the terrible human rights conditions south of the border. I presented papers in academic meetings and wrote articles analyzing the forces responsible for the human rights debacle occurring in the Southern Cone. Along with many colleagues in the interdisciplinary field of Latin American Studies, I was especially committed to analyzing the hegemonic role the US played in the repression of much-needed social change throughout the region. Toward this end, we organized the Latin American solidarity movement on campuses and among trade unions in this country in support of peoples' struggles. One of the most difficult aspects of this period was my emotional experience of disaffection from people in this country who, beyond the Latin American academic and solidarity community, knew little and, I resentfully believed, cared less about what was happening in their name beyond our national borders. I traversed two very different realities, and the distance between the two often produced feelings of helpless rage toward my compatriots. I believed their disinterest was responsible for the escalating violence against people I knew and loved who were rapidly becoming targets of a ruthless military onslaught financially, diplomatically and militarily supported by the US government and corporate elites. Among those people was Carlos Perez, a book publisher with whom I had been in a relationship for several of those tumultuous years (Feitlowitz, 1998).

Once the coup occurred on March 20, 1976, I was not able to return to Argentina. As the armed forces invaded all facets of life, they took aim against ideas as well as individuals and groups they deemed enemies of "Western Christian civilization." In the process, a book I had published in Buenos Aires in 1974 called *Women: History of Slaves or Slaves of History*? (Hollander, 1974), was among the thousands of books burned in the streets by the fascist-identified military determined to kill off all critical thinking that threatened their domination over Argentine society.

I had little idea at the time that these experiences represented for me a cumulative traumatic wound that was unrecognized as such and thus left unattended. I had even less understanding of their connection to earlier traumatic experiences that, as a child and adolescent, I had struggled to manage alone, often by turning to poetry and literature as solace and a way of finding meaning and connection to others who were able to express much of what was inchoate in my own awareness of self. This interest in internal states and relational experience had originally led me to choose psychology as an undergraduate major. One psychology course I took required a practicum, and I elected to work in a state-subsidized daycare center for working-class parents, where I took care of the children until their parents arrived in the early evening to pick them up. Repeatedly I witnessed how the overwrought and exhausted parents responded with impatience and irritation to their toddlers' eager need for recognition and connection after a long day's separation. My (not yet analyzed) associations to my own early struggles with a narcissistically preoccupied mother and the early loss of my father to cancer made the nightly ritual agonizing. My identification with the emotionally neglected and agitated children was so disturbing that my observant advisor suggested I choose another career until I could work through the issues that were making the experience so burdensome for me. She did not speak about transference, but her advice felt like a welcome release, and the next semester I switched my major to history. That field presented similar themes of power/victimization and authority/submission. As an historian I could address some of the same dynamics I saw in the daycare center, only now in a broadly contextualized and less personally painful way because they could be thought about in the context of large group dynamics occurring over the course of hundreds of years. Further, I could experience a kind of vicarious gratification that came from studying the multiple historical examples of individuals and groups who were able to fight to overturn the authorities and conditions that oppressed them. But this intellectual resolution turned out to be chimerical, given the particular history I would ultimately choose to specialize in and then to live!

And, in the end, I found my way back to psychology. A precipitating event in this regard occurred when I went to Madrid in the summer of 1981 with the purpose of interviewing a number of Argentine women who had fled into exile to escape the military state and its torturers. One woman told of having to abandon her children to relatives as she frantically scrambled to elude the military forces stalking her from house to house; another revealed how, as she walked along the wide avenues of Buenos Aires, she was kidnapped by hooded men leaping out at her from one of the infamous unmarked Ford Falcons used by the right-wing death squads. Ultimately she was left for dead on a remote country road after being tortured and raped in one of the government's clandestine concentration camps. Another woman spoke of having been sought by military forces who, bursting into her home without a warrant and finding only her younger brother, kidnapped him instead, torturing and killing him for no reason in particular. Yet another told of being forced to watch while prison guards tortured her elderly parents in order to secure information she did not have; and one reported how, when her pregnant daughter suddenly vanished, clearly the victim of a military or death-squad action, her endless searches for her daughter and grandchild yielded nothing but a gaping hole in her heart; many told of having narrowly escaped similar fates before they were forced to flee into the uncertainty and dislocation of exile.

As I listened, I was aware of how important it was to these women that they could offer testimony about their life-shattering experiences. Bearing witness was excruciating but crucial for me as well, even though I felt overtaken by a sense of profound horror. And I realized I could not depend on my social science training or my radical political theory or my feminist analysis to understand these women as individual survivors of a collective tragedy. I could not account for their capacity to endure the brutalities to which they had been subjected without going mad. Nor could I explain the variation in their success or failure to cope psychologically with such severe life disruptions and losses. Not present, but like ghosts, were the torturers themselves and, for me at the time, their equally inexplicable capacity to inflict such sadistic assaults on the minds and bodies of fellow human beings. I had not yet learned to think in terms of trauma and traumatogenic triggers that can constitute a veritable undoing of the psyche, nor in terms of the psychology of the perpetrator and its relationship to trauma. Only when I was subsequently introduced to psychoanalytic theory and clinical experience would I come to understand that the differences I noted in these survivors, which could be accounted for by individual psychodynamics and the diverse consequences and meanings made of traumatic experience, nonetheless, hid what was shared in common: the endurable wounds of having encountered the Lacanian Real (Zizek, 1989, 2002; Boulanger, 2007).

Psychoanalysis, trauma, and politics

When I first met Austrian-born Argentine psychoanalyst Marie Langer in the early 1980s, I was a Professor of Latin American history and Gender Studies, and my familiarity with psychoanalytic theory came through the lens of feminist writers' reinterpretation of object relations and Lacanian theories. While by then I was in a personal psychoanalysis and married to Steve Portuges, a psychologist in psychoanalytic training whose social radicalism paralleled my own, psychoanalysis was not yet integrated into my political life, which still revolved around the Latin American solidarity movements. I was producing and hosting a bi-weekly hour-long program on Pacifica Radio, for which I interviewed Latin America scholars and activists—among whom were feminist intellectuals and organizers—whose experience and analyses could enlighten the US public about the political realities throughout the region. One of these individuals sent me a copy of Marie Langer's recently published book that described her life as a politically radical psychoanalyst in Argentina because, as he presciently told me, I would find much in common with her (Langer, 1981). As I read it, I became enthralled with the woman who emerged from its pages and knew at once that I wanted to write her biography. Her life embraced the three most important modes of thought of the twentieth century—Marxism, feminism and psychoanalysis—in the context of some of the century's most tumultuous social conditions. With that goal in mind, I contacted her, not realizing how much our relationship would dramatically change and enrich my life.

Langer, one of the six founders of the prestigious Argentine Psychoanalytic Association and among Latin America's most prominent psychoanalysts, was then in her mid-seventies and living in Mexico City, along with thousands of other Argentines forced into exile. She had been a major figure among the psychoanalysts in Argentina who, during the same period I had been there, had responded to the turbulent social and political conditions by developing a theoretical orientation that integrated object relations and Lacanian ideas with radical social theory, and which they practiced in an activism that aligned them with human rights and social justice movements. They had ventured out of their offices located in the bourgeois neighborhoods of Buenos Aires to bring their clinical services to poor and working-class communities and to the victims of military and police repression as well. In 1974, as political polarization intensified and paramilitary forces operated quite openly, Langer was forced to flee Argentina into exile after being told by a patient that she had been targeted for assassination by the infamous death squad, the Argentine Anticommunist Alliance. In Mexico, she was rapidly integrated into the Mexican psychoanalytic community, but her passions lay with the solidarity work among refugees from the Southern Cone and increasingly from the bloody civil wars encompassing Central America. She treated victims of imprisonment and torture among the refugee populations and, most importantly, by the time I met her she was the ecstatically enthusiastic Co-coordinator of the Internationalist Team of Mental Health Workers, Mexico-Nicaragua, whose purpose was to help the Sandinista Revolution develop Nicaragua's first national mental health care system.

When I proposed the biographical project to her, I was stunned by her immediate agreement, not realizing that she already knew me through my film, *Communiqué from Argentina*, which she had seen several years earlier when my co-director and I were invited to screen it for the exile community in the Argentine Center in Mexico City. Thus I was welcomed into the world of "Mimi" Langer, and my psychoanalytic education began. Through Mimi I met a network of colleagues, mainly from Argentina, but also from Uruguay, Chile, Brazil and Mexico, who provided an important bridge for my own integration of social and psychological theory and political activism. Their example led me to seek my own psychoanalytic training in Los Angeles. Over the years, my relationship with my Latin American colleagues has enriched my theoretical and clinical understanding of how social trauma operates, often silently, as a pathogen that corrodes subjective and interpersonal relations, the symptoms of which can be decoded by a psychoanalytic method that takes account of the social matrix of psychic malaise. Thus the customary emphasis on the familial-based etiology of psychological disorders can be situated in the larger social context of ideological and institutional structuring of unconscious processes and intersubjective experience. This orientation has guided my research and writing on the psychological impact of social trauma in the context of the state terrorist regimes and the nominally democratic cultures of impunity that succeeded them in the Southern Cone.

I was able to spend considerable time with Mimi while she lived in Mexico City, where I traveled frequently to visit and record almost 60 hours of interviews for my biographical project about her life and work. As well, I interviewed her and other Latin American mental health professionals for my radio program so that they could speak about their experiences and psychoanalytically informed understanding of the psychological impact of political repression and exile, with the inevitable sequelae among survivors of what Mimi called "frozen grief." Most importantly, I was present several times when the Internationalist Team of Mental Health Workers held their inviolable Monday evening meetings in Mimi's home. During these meetings I learned about their objectives, pedagogical and clinical methodologies and their resolution of the challenges to sustain continuity in their work in Nicaragua. Each month two members of the team's 12 psychoanalysts, psychiatrists and psychologists went on a rotating basis to Nicaragua for 10 days to teach and train their counterparts in the underdeveloped conditions of that tiny, impoverished Central American nation. The Sandinista Revolution had just overthrown the repressive US-supported Somoza dictatorship and was developing sweeping reforms, including a mixed state and private sector economic model, a parliament composed of representatives of multiple political parties and mass-based popular organizations and a nonaligned foreign policy.

Mimi's enthusiasm for this work was contagious, and I came to agree with her that it was a unique chapter in the history of psychoanalysis as it offered an opportunity to actualize in practice the Freud–Marx discourse: here was a revolutionary government with a commitment to building the country's first mental health care system based in psychoanalytic concepts and clinical methods. When I traveled to Nicaragua with Mimi and Ignacio (Nacho) Maldonado in the summer of 1983, I was to see firsthand the range of their creative contributions to the country's efforts to deal with the collective traumatic legacy of decades of dictatorship and years of revolutionary struggle. Moreover, additional psychological challenges occurred in response to the Revolution's commitment to reform traditional class and gender relations. In a unique way, psychoanalysis was setting down roots in the fertile soil of a society committed to social democracy and a radical restructuring of power hierarchies. The Internationalist Team taught theory and clinical technique, carefully adapted to the particular economic and cultural conditions of Nicaragua, to psychiatrists and social workers in Managua's only psychiatric hospital, to physicians and medical students at the University of Leon and to the psychologists and social workers in the burgeoning community mental health clinics being established throughout the country. They also supervised mental health professionals who worked with the various mass organizations that mobilized different sectors of the Nicaraguan population—women, peasants, students, refugees from neighboring El Salvador and Guatemala—who were then collectively able to represent their sectoral interests. I eagerly absorbed the important lessons of this experience (Langer and Maldonado, 1983). To my Argentine colleagues, whose prior efforts at utilizing their psychoanalytic expertise beyond the couch had occurred in politically repressive circumstances in which the state was aligned against them, Nicaragua represented the possibility of being able to join with others in the construction of a new future, one that took seriously the provision of resources and social bonds of support and solidarity conducive to personal development. As I witnessed their clinical work in these various settings, I was learning how to understand the convergences between individual psychologies and collectively shared trauma. I also had the opportunity to observe my teachers' management of transference and countertransference dynamics as they occurred in light of each unique dyadic encounter as well as the passionate reactions for and against the very political process that made access to mental health care and these mental health professionals a human right. Just as it did for me, I knew that for Mimi and Nacho Nicaragua represented a reparative experience given their respective and shared histories of loss, unresolved mourning and guilt at having survived Argentine state terror when others had not.

Mimi Langer did not live to see the end of this psychoanalytic experiment after President Reagan's low-intensity war strategy (Klare and Kornbluh, 1998) and the Nicaraguan elites succeeded in ousting the Sandinistas in the 1990 elections. Mimi died of inoperable cancer in December 1987. She was publicly eulogized in intellectual and psychoanalytic circles from Argentina to Vienna; her death was devastating to those who knew and loved her. She had been my mentor, and, in a variety of ways, the good mother I had never had, as well as my infant son's adopted grandmother. My friendships with the younger generation of psychoanalysts for whom she had been an inspiration, and who had participated with her in shared political struggles, provided an essential means by which I could maintain coherence with a psychoanalytic paradigm I had come to embrace through my experiences with Mimi.

Since Mimi's death I have returned often to the Southern Cone in order to study and write about the psychological sequelae of the region's state terrorist regimes, whose repressive policies included the disappearing, torturing and murdering of tens of thousands of civilians. I studied the cultures of impunity imposed by subsequent governments, in which survivors of human rights abuses experienced retraumatization because of the lack of effective accountability of former perpetrators. Impunity included not only freedom for torturers but the imposition of a social agenda based on a globalized neoliberal agenda. The consequent worsening of the very inequitable social and economic conditions that the prior era's radical movements had fought against produced a collective demoralization. Many of my psychoanalytic colleagues have continued to develop social projects that combine theoretical analysis and psychotherapeutic interventions for the direct and indirect victims of state terror and for those who have suffered the multiple assaults of corrupt democratic governments. In so doing, they continue to maintain a critical social psychoanalytic presence in myriad progressive struggles for social change. For example, in response to the traumatic impact of the complete economic collapse in Argentina in December 2001, a network of psychoanalysts contributed in innovative ways to help foster resilience in the face of terrifying threats to survival. Argentine citizens mobilized grassroots movements that took over their communities to run them themselves. In response to the scarcity of money as a means of exchange, they created huge flea markets in which neighbors bartered goods and services among themselves as a collective survival strategy. Neighbors participated in spontaneous community meetings in the streets to discuss what to do with their decimated economy and incompetent government (Hollander, 2004). Workers took over factories abandoned by owners who had fled the country with their capital and other assets and collectively figured out how to operate and administer the production and distribution processes without their bosses. Psychoanalysts participated in these social movements and, where they could, brought their psychological and other support skills to aid those suffering from anxieties of all kinds provoked by a traumatogenic social environment. Especially in the occupied factories, psychoanalysts contributed to the efforts of workers as they faced unprecedented work challenges at the same time as they had to organize resources for their daily survival. These analysts practiced a "psychoanalysis without the couch" as they met informally with workers in the factories' hallways or cafeterias at unpredictable hours, providing invaluable interventions with the women and men living in the factories who needed therapeutic help to deal with the intrapsychic and interpersonal conflicts triggered by their revolutionary challenge to the ideological pillars of political authority and private property. This type of socially committed work has continued in multiple ways in Argentina and elsewhere in the region and constitutes an important chapter in the history of Latin American psychoanalysis. I have been inspired by its example and have written extensively about what I believe to be an important social psychoanalytic model that like-minded psychoanalysts in other countries may be able to adapt to their own specific sociopolitical environments (Hollander, 2010a).

In my own work, I have attempted to integrate social theory and psychoanalytic concepts to understand what I have lived through and witnessed, first by applying object relations theory and later by incorporating relational theory as well as concepts derived from the British group psychotherapy and Lacanian traditions. By the mid-1990s, my social psychoanalytic frame originally developed in the context of the extreme social situation of Latin America permitted me to see and write about the less obvious but eerily similar patterns that were emerging in the social, political and economic trends in this country, with disquieting psychological implications for citizens in the heart of Empire (Hollander, 2007, pp. 163–191). Since 9/11, I have analyzed the complex trauma involved in the loss of American exceptionalism and its concomitant features of political authoritarianism and economic implosion that have borne heavily on the psychological experience of the citizens of this country. I have striven to develop a theoretical approach that integrates social and psychological theory in an exploration of socially created subjectivities whose unconscious fantasies, affects and defenses are shaped by the hegemonic cultural symbols of the social order's asymmetrical forces of privilege and power (Hollander, 2010a, 2010b).

I feel fortunate to have found a network of psychoanalytic colleagues in the US with whom I share a commitment to psychoanalysis and social responsibility. Indeed, the psychoanalytic community in this country has provided me the opportunity to speak and write about the interface between social and psychic reality in both Latin America and the US. As with all victims of trauma, I have experienced a kind of reparative healing in the experience of being heard and of finding resonance among colleagues whose preoccupations mirror my own. Over time, this sense of community has diminished the deeply disturbing split I felt years ago when I found little responsiveness in most circles to the social trauma I witnessed and experienced south of the border.

In fact, it was my work on Marie Langer that prompted Susan Gutwill, a graduate of the feminist psychoanalytic Women's Therapy Center Institute, to contact me to learn more about the practice of Latin American psychoanalysis under extreme social conditions. This transcontinental phone call turned out to be the initiation of a years-long intellectual and writing collaboration and the first of many important relationships that I went on to develop through organizations such as Psychoanalysis for Social Responsibility (Section 9 of the Division of Psychoanalysis, American Psychological Association (APA)), the Association for Psychoanalysis, Culture and Society and the Los Angeles-based Uprooted Mind Committee that has organized many community events focusing on psychoanalytic perspectives on living in a dangerous world. These colleagues, who are committed to a psychoanalysis that is identified with principles of social justice, have provided a North American home for me, one that resonates with the values and principles I have found so profoundly important in Latin America. One meaningful intellectual project emerged from presentations over several years on panels organized for Division 39 meetings by Section 9, which Lynne Layton, Susan Gutwill and I edited into a volume called *Psychoanalysis, Class and Politics: Encounters in the Clinical Setting* (2006). Another important experience I had, along with other members of Section 9, was our participation in the struggle to challenge and reform the APA's Ethics policy that had permitted psychologists to engage in the government's enhanced interrogations of detainees at Guantánamo and elsewhere (Reisner, 2010). This effort resonated with what I have written about my Latin American colleagues' struggles to expose and prohibit the participation of mental health professionals in the torture policies of their authoritarian governments (Hollander, 2011). Another experience that has provided me with a profound sense of continuity has been my decade-long membership in the Psychoanalytic Work Group for Peace in Palestine/Israel, composed of ten North American Arab and Jewish psychoanalysts, Palestinian and Jewish Israeli psychoanalysts and psychoanalytically oriented Palestinian psychologists. This unique group applies psychoanalytic thinking to the complex dynamics of the "intractable struggle" and has organized symposia and dialogues with the goal of facilitating and modeling empathic understanding among groups in conflict.

As I think about the complex implications of Laplanche's concept of "afterwardsness," it is clear to me that my childhood and adult experiences with traumatic loss (tinged with survival guilt) are continually reworked in the light of shifting conflicts and gratifications in the present. They simultaneously inform present anxieties that get stirred up by my interest in—and perhaps preoccupation with—the deepening political crises that foment individual and group psychological distress. The past also shadows my adaptive efforts at reparation, lending a doggedly passionate commitment to the paradigm of a social psychoanalysis that I believe can help shed light on the dynamics of human destructiveness and contribute to strategies that facilitate capacities for caring, resilience and empathic connection. While I have explored and refined clinical technique throughout my career, from my perspective, given the increasingly incontrovertible traumatic stressors stemming from the social world that impinge on our most intimate psychological experience, I can best make my contribution to psychoanalysis in this country by continuing to think and write about the mutual impact of social forces and hegemonic ideology on the one hand and intrapsychic and intersubjective dynamics on the other.

I said earlier that politics had led me to psychoanalysis and that psychoanalysis can deepen our understanding of the political psyche. I believe that the current conditions produced by negative globalization are fostering what Zygmunt Bauman has called "liquid fears" (Bauman, 2007), by which he means rapidly cycling terrors that attach themselves to any number of global threats, moving from economic implosion to climate change to terrorism to pandemic diseases and on and on. From my perspective, these socially produced traumatogenic features of our world are a legitimate concern of psychoanalysis, both as essential aspects of our theory as well as a focus of clinical attention as they emerge more or less silently, often invisible to both analyst and patient when they are not considered to be an appropriate subject of psychoanalytic attention. My therapeutic work with survivors of torture and losses of loved ones perpetrated by state terrorist regimes has trained me to be vigilantly aware of how socially induced traumatic symptoms may be experienced by patients—and ourselves—in response to the destabilizing and multiplying crises produced by the increasingly threatening economic and political conditions in this country and the world. From my perspective, we live in times that call for a socially responsible psychoanalysis, one that finds common cause with the radical origins of our profession.

In this sense, the Occupy movement, with which I began this personal narrative, represents the ability of people to emerge from an identification (largely unconscious) with hegemony toward a more (conscious) critical subjectivity. For all its contradictory characteristics, the Occupy movement has created an alternative discourse to the prevailing ideological justifications of our own culture of impunity. From my perspective, its value, beyond its immediate fate as a political force in this country, resides in its symbolic significance of the human capacity for resilience in the face of trauma.

As a psychoanalyst, I believe our profession can enrich our understanding of the dynamic processes that potentiate these capacities in people. As a political activist, I support a psychoanalysis beyond the couch, one that is engaged in reparative efforts to reform the socially traumatic conditions that are creating the collective malaise of our times.

Note

1 Reprinted from *Psychoanalysis, Culture & Society, suppl. Special Issue: Psychoanalysis, Trauma, and Community* 18.2 (Jun 2013): 167–183 by permission of Palgrave Macmillan.

References

Bauman, Z. (2007) *Liquid Fear*. Cambridge: Polity Press.

Blumenkranz, C. Gessen, K., Greif, M., Leonard, S., Resnick, S., Saval, N., Schmitt, E. and Taylor, N. (2011) *Occupy!: Scenes from Occupied America*. London: Verso.

Boggs, C. (1984) *The Two Revolutions: Antonio Gramsci and the Dilemmas of Western Marxism*. Cambridge: South End Press.

Boulanger, G. (2007) *Wounded by Reality: Understanding and Treating Adult Onset Trauma*. Mahwah: Analytic Press.

Bray, M.W. (2012) The Making of Chile: With Poems and Guns: A personal recollection. http://lap.sagepub.com/search/results?fulltext=Chile%3A+With+Poems+and+Guns&x=13&y=8&submit=yes&journal_set=splap&src=selected&andorexactfulltext=and online or LAP, accessed August 2, 2012.

Damousi, J. and Plotkin, M.B. (eds) (2012) *Psychoanalysis and Politics*. New York: Oxford University Press.

Feitlowitz, M. (1998) *A Lexicon of Terror: Argentina and the Legacies of Torture*. New York: Oxford University Press.

Gitlin, T. (2012) *Occupy Nation: The Roots, the Spirit, and the Promise of Occupy Wall Street*. New York: It Books.

Harris, A. and Botticelli, S. (2010) *First Do No Harm: The Paradoxical Encounters of Psychoanalysis, Warmaking, and Resistance.* New York: Routledge.

Hollander, N.C. (1974) *La mujer: esclava de la historia o historia de esclava?* Buenos Aires: La Pléyade.

Hollander, N.C. (1990) Buenos Aires, Argentina: Latin Mecca of psychoanalysis. *Social Research* 57 (4): 889–919.

Hollander, N.C. (editor of special issue) (2004) Argentine economic meltdown: Trauma and social resistance. *Mind and Human Interaction* 13 (4): 161–238.

Hollander, N.C. (2007) *Love in a Time of Hate: Liberation Psychology in Latin America*. New York: Other Books.

Hollander, N.C. (2010a) *Uprooted Minds: Surviving the Politics of Terror in the Americas*. New York: Routledge.

Hollander, N.C. (2010b) The gendering of human rights: Women and the Latin American terrorist state. In: A. Harris and S. Botticelli (eds) *First Do No Harm: The Paradoxical Encounters of Psychoanalysis, Warmaking, and Resistance*. New York: Routledge, pp. 279–301.

Hollander, N.C. (2011) Psycho-political dynamics of the bystander in Luis Puenzo's "The official story." Special issue: Witnessing, hiding, bystanding—Contributions from film to their social consequences. *International Journal of Applied Psychoanalytic Studies* 8 (2): 147–161.

Jacoby, R. (1983) *The Repression of Psychoanalysis: Otto Fenichel and the Freudians*. New York: Basic Books.

Klare, M. and Kornbluh, P. (eds) (1998) *Low Intensity Warfare: Counterinsurgency, Proinsurgency and Antiterrorism in the Eighties*. New York: Pantheon Books.

Langer, M. (1971) Psícoanalisis y/O revolución social. *Cuestionamos I*: 261–284.

Langer, M. (1981) *Memoria, historia y diálogo psicoanalítico*. Mexico City: Folios Ediciones.

Langer, M. and Maldonado, I. (1983) Unpublished manuscript.

Layton, L., Hollander, N.C. and Gutwill, S. (eds) (2006) *Psychoanalysis, Class and Politics: Encounters in the Clinical Setting*. New York: Routledge.
Laplanche, J. (1999a) *Essays on Otherness*. New York: Routledge.
Laplanche, J. (1999b) *The Unconscious and the Id*. London: Rebus Press.
Reisner, S. (2010) From resistance to *resistance*: A narrative of psychoanalytic activism. In: A. Harris and S. Botticelli (eds) *First Do No Harm: The Paradoxical Encounters of Psychoanalysis, Warmaking, and Resistance*. New York: Routledge, pp. 107–141.
Zizek, S. (1989) *The Sublime Object of Ideology*. London: Verso.
Zizek, S. (2002) *Welcome to the Desert of the Real*. London: Verso.

Chapter 12

Institutional betrayal and the case of the American Psychological Association

The role of psychoanalysts and psychoanalysis in challenging it

Elizabeth Hegeman

What can the members of a professional organization expect from it? What do the employees of a national organization owe to its members? These questions have special importance in the light of the recent Hoffman report (2015) detailing the history of "collusion" (in the report's terms) between American Psychological Association (APA) senior leadership and the military intelligence community. At the same time the senior leadership was publicly condemning torture, it put forth deceptive public relations claims that falsely portrayed APA as concerned with the welfare of detainees.

This chapter will explore the relationship between the members of the APA and the administration/governance of the APA, and it will focus on the role of some members of the APA and of Division 39, the Division of Psychoanalysis, in their attempts to influence policy and actions of the organization as a whole. The facts presented are based mostly on the abovementioned Hoffman report, an independent report commissioned in November 2014 by Nadine Kaslow, Ph.D., and the Committee for the Independent Review of allegations of collusion in response to *New York Times* reporter James Risen's (2014) book, *Pay Any Price: Greed, Power and Endless War*. The Hoffman report was written by a team of six lawyers working with David Hoffman of the Sidley Austin law firm in Chicago, who examined many years of documents and emails from within and between the APA and other organizations such as the US government, especially the Department of Defense (DOD) and the Central Intelligence Agency (CIA).

Like many others, I became active within Section 9 (Social Responsibility) of Division 39 of the APA in organizing and protesting when APA involvement with the military became public in 2006; I subsequently resigned from APA in 2009 in protest when it was clear that the 2008 Referendum enjoining psychologists' participation in interrogations would not be implemented, despite having been passed by a majority of the membership. I continued to follow developments by reading news stories, communications, and reports from Division 39's Section 9 and Section 56 (Trauma). Other psychologists and psychoanalysts continued to work within the APA to bring about change in policies regarding interrogation and with the organization itself. For further perspective, I interviewed by telephone Laurel Bass Wagner, Ph.D., who served on the APA Council for six years, and corresponded by email in January 2015 with Ghislaine Boulanger, Ph.D., who first suggested the tactic of withholding dues.

A brief history of the issues

Psychoanalysts have played a key role in opposing the participation of psychologists in torture and interrogation at Guantanamo Bay and other illegal detention sites. The principles and experience of psychoanalysts treating victims of trauma intensively may have sensitized them to these issues and moved them to act as change agents to influence other psychologists to become active in insisting that ethics rules be restored and enforced. While the recent (August 2015) resolution of the Council of Representatives of APA, which prohibits psychologists' participation in interrogations, is gratifying to some (Vasquez, 2016), the full implications of the Hoffman report have yet to be addressed. It is clear that this resolution, and others from various offices and committees of APA that preceded it, do not have the binding enforceability that changes in the ethics code would have (Pope, 2016). It is likely that without continued efforts from dedicated people inside and outside the organization to bring APA action in line with its stated policy (Risen, 2015), attention to issues of torture and interrogation might never have found continued and growing public support from recent investigative reporters (Risen, 2014) and congressional hearings (Feinstein, 2014). The full history of strenuous efforts made by psychologists and psychoanalyst–psychologists to try to bring about an honorable response, and the continued deception of APA leadership, has been documented in books (Harris and Botticelli, 2010), on several websites (e.g., www.ethicalpsychology.com) and in documentary films (www.MarthaDavis.com), and most recently, in the Hoffman report, in a move toward transparency.

Institutional betrayal

In September 2014, the *American Psychologist*, the monthly publication of the APA, published an article entitled "Institutional Betrayal." The authors, Carly Smith and Jennifer Freyd, defined institutional betrayal as "trusted and powerful institutions (schools, churches, military, government) acting in ways that visit harm upon those dependent on them for safety and well-being" (p. 575), and stated that their purpose was

> to describe psychological research that examines the role of institutions in traumatic experiences and psychological distress following these experiences. We demonstrate the ways in which institutional betrayal has been left unseen by both the individuals being betrayed as well as the field of psychology and introduce means by which to identify and address this betrayal. (p. 575)

The cases they discussed include a suicide by a college freshman whose report of sexual abuse was met with harassment and insensitive investigative practices; childhood sexual abuse by clergy, coaches, and teachers; and members of the armed services who were punished for reporting sexual abuse. Smith and Freyd relied heavily on relational psychoanalytic principles in describing their theory. They developed a strong parallel between institutional and individual relational betrayal in close personal relationships and the traumatic consequences of each. They pointed out that institutions normally foster a sense of trust and/or dependency, and they described typical institutional reactions and patterns of denial when the betrayal is uncovered, which fit the facts and history of the APA non-reaction to member protests and reports of ethics violations. However, Smith and Freyd did not mention or discuss the APA's betrayal of its members who have tried to influence the organization to enforce its own ethics principles in reference to interrogation procedures at Guantanamo Bay and other illegal military detention sites. Despite the release of the Hoffman report, and because of the processes of denial and dissociation described in the article and in this chapter, this failure is probably not widely enough understood by the membership or by the public at large.

According to Philip Zimbardo (2008), people are influenced to wrongdoing and misuse of power by group and contextual factors, not just individual moral factors. Zimbardo conducted the Stanford Prison Experiment, in which undergraduates simulated the roles of prisoners and guards; the experiment had to be stopped early because the "guards" had become so brutal after six days (and the inmates so symptomatic) that Zimbardo and his staff were afraid of the effects on the volunteer subjects. This research is useful for us to understand not only the behavior of the prison guards at Abu Ghraib and Guantanamo Bay, but also the behavior and decisions of some office holders and decision makers within the APA. Zimbardo believes that under the right conditions, anyone can commit atrocities; many social psychology experiments have demonstrated how easy it is to turn a deaf ear or a blind eye to harm being done to others, and even to participate as an actor in certain contexts (Milgram, 1983). What happened in APA from 2002–2015 was a complex social phenomenon involving dynamics of power, money, and status, not something that could be attributed only to a guilty few or limited to a single part of an organization.

Dissociation and betrayal

Many members of the APA struggled to oppose the organization's collusion with the CIA and military interests, without visible impact, especially between 2006 and the present. This illustrates Smith and Freyd's definition of institutional betrayal and the effects of the APA's policies on professional psychoanalysts and psychologists. I will examine possible reasons why some were not "blinded" to the betrayal and how many others continue to dissociate from the harm done by the APA's covert opposition to enforcement of the ethics code.

Psychoanalysis and psychoanalysts are concerned with understanding and analyzing unconscious and conscious motivation and are accustomed to applying concepts such as identification with the aggressor, sadism, masochism, narcissism, and especially dissociation (a defense by not seeing or realizing something threatening) to human behavior. Psychoanalysts have also been active in treating the victims of human aggression and in disseminating an understanding of lasting psychic harm from cruelty. These factors influenced many of those who spearheaded opposition to the negligence and secret collusion of the APA with the CIA, the DOD, and the US military, as they were professionally dedicated to thinking about and noticing unconscious and disavowed aggression.

Torture and the professions

For Smith and Freyd (2014), publishing this essay in an organ of the APA illustrates the authors' central point that "institutional betrayal has been left unseen by both the individuals being betrayed as well as (unseen by) the field of psychology" (p. 577). Betrayal trauma within a trusted relationship is associated with more severe emotional consequences than other forms of betrayal, in part because the coping strategy required for preservation of the relationship requires "extended unawareness or 'blindness' to the betrayal trauma" (p. 577). The most egregious betrayal perpetrated by the APA, both of its members and of the public trust, has to do with its failure to take effective action against the current and past participation of psychologists in the design and carrying out of torture of prisoners not only in Guantanamo Bay, but in all of the "black sites" where prisoners are held in violation of United Nations (UN) guidelines and the Geneva conventions. Since 2001, psychology alone among the professions has allowed itself and its name to be used to legitimize inhuman treatment of prisoners. All of the other professions dedicated to human care—such as the American Medical Association, American Bar Association, American Psychiatric Association, and American Counseling Association—have not only explicitly abjured participation in torture, but have also incorporated language and examples in their codes of ethics to allow for enforcement. But the psychologists who designed and carried out the military's Behavioral Sciences Consultation Team (BSCT) program and the reverse-engineered Survival, Evasion, Resistance and Escape (SERE) tactics have allowed themselves to be used in order to give the appearance of professional approval to these practices, at the expense of the humiliation and degradation of the field of psychology in the eyes of the American public and the world. The APA's inaction in enforcing ethical principles and its covert attempts to obtain a favored position with the agencies conducting interrogations illustrates Smith and Freyd's definition of institutional betrayal and its harm to the profession of psychology.

Theory: what can we learn from what happened?

We could invoke psychodynamic theory to attempt to explain this institutional behavior: Was it idealization of governance by the membership? Or, as some might say, was it regressive transference to leaders, in hopes of finding a good parent? Was it denial, inattention, and ignorance on the part of the membership? A few bad apples? All these explanations pathologize and tend to shift blame onto individuals or a small group, which misses the more important process of social construction of values and behavior. We need a more comprehensive theory, one that does more than single out individuals to blame.

An interesting clue could come from the data of the lawsuit brought against the APA Practice Organization, the companion organization to the APA, which supports the mechanics of professional practice. Beginning in 2006, this lawsuit had to survive many defeats and legal appeals; unlike the ethics complaints, however, it has finally succeeded. This year, the US District Court of the District of Columbia found that the Practice Directorate—although admitting no wrongdoing—had misled members into thinking that a fee was mandatory when it was not. As a result, $9.2 million in refunds and damages were ordered to be repaid to members. Was this suit (and the concentrated effort it required) a reverberation of members' dissatisfaction and suspicion, a blip of the felt sense of betrayal, displaced onto a more trivial and self-interested issue than torture? How do we account for the success of this lawsuit where ethics complaints to national associations and state boards failed?

There is a deeper problem here, one that goes beyond wrongdoing. It is a concept that psychoanalysts should be thoroughly familiar with—the problem of unconscious bias and social construction. Nancy Hollander (2014) has described in detail how existing power arrangements in a society come to be normalized and internalized, contributing to the sense of rightness and belonging.

> The social unconscious includes the installation of power relations within the core of psychic structure that functions as a bridge between the group and the individual to shape drives, affects and defenses … On the one hand it enables individuals to acquire a coherent self-image that covers over the original state of decenteredness characteristic of early life. But it also creates subjects who uncritically identify with the social order's repressive and constraining asymmetrical relations of authority and power (p. 5).

As Hollander has stated so well, the very process of individuation for each person requires the internalization of the realities of power in the social group in which we live. It is completely natural not to question authority; in fact a successful childrearing process means to accept the rules and positions of power we have come to know. So the members of the organization and its elected representatives (although not necessarily its paid employees, as I will discuss later) naturally respect and trust its decisions.

A history of APA ethics codes

One of the hallmarks of a profession is the right to police and regulate the actions of its members. Professions are expected to maintain codes of ethics and enforce ethical practices. APA members complained for years, especially from 2002 to the present, when the organization made no response to ethics complaints (see www.ethicalpsychology.org). Ken Pope, former ethics director, reported that as early as the 1990s, the APA "had turned away from its responsibility to protect the public" (2015, pp. 148–150). Post-9/11 violations have been the focus of recent protest; the Hoffman report (2015) quotes the most recent APA ethics director's statement that the role of APA ethics "is not protection of the public and that protection of the public is a function for state licensing boards" (p. 475). But according to Pope (2016), this crucial shift in the code took place much earlier: "APA's initial move away from protecting the public sparked great controversy with publication of the 1992 Ethics code." He quotes Don Bersoff, former general counsel and later president of APA, as saying "the code is full of such lawyer-driven 'weasel words' as reasonable and feasible" (Pope 2016, p. 366). Thus, according to Pope and Hoffman, the shift toward protection of psychologists rather than the public dates back to the code changes of 1992.

We have only learned gradually of the active role played by APA in seeking a special role as consultants in interrogation. In fact, these realities—brought out by Stephen Soldz, Stephen Reisner, and others—might still be buried in websites but for James Risen (2014), a reporter for the *New York Times*, in *Pay Any Price: Greed, Power and Endless War*. He states on the basis of email evidence that the president of APA reached out to the CIA as early as December 2001. According to www.ethicalpsychology.org, a crucial change to Principle 1.02 of the Ethics Code was adopted by the Council of Representatives on August 21, 2002, to allow psychologists to defer to legal authorities if an ethical conflict between professional ethics code and a direct order could not be resolved "in a responsible manner." This position—often referred to as the "Nuremberg Defense"—allows a person to say "I was only following orders" as a legal defense. This change was commonly attributed to a reaction to the events of 9/11, although the Hoffman report found that discussion of the change in wording predated 9/11. The 2002 wording reads:

> If psychologists' ethical responsibilities conflict with law, regulations, or other governing legal authority, then psychologists make known their commitment to (this) Ethics Code and take steps to resolve the conflict in a responsible manner. If the conflict is unresolvable via such means, psychologists may adhere to the requirements of the law, regulations, or other governing authority in keeping with basic principles of human rights.
>
> (APA website, p. 3 of comparison of 1992 and 2002 Ethics Codes)

The earlier 1992 code did not give explicit permission to psychologists to follow the legal order:

> If the Ethics Code standard appears to conflict with the requirements of law, then psychologists make known their commitment to the Ethics Code and take steps to resolve the conflict in a responsible manner. If neither law nor the Ethics Code resolves an issue, psychologists should consider other professional materials and the dictates of their own conscience, as well as seek consultation with others within the field when this is practical.
>
> (ibid., APA website, p. 3)

Although even the Hoffman report acknowledges that these changes although approved in 2002 were in the works much earlier, the crucial change which gives permission to psychologists to "adhere to the requirements of the law, regulations, or other governing authority" was the basis for APA's ability to maneuver for psychologists to contract with DOD and participate in interrogations.

Although the positions and actions of the Bush Administration regarding interrogations were to some extent public, the complex behind-the-scenes involvement of the APA in the attempt to carve out a role for psychologists in interrogation did not begin to become fully apparent to the membership until a few members reacted to the secrecy and manipulation of the Psychological Ethics and National Security (PENS) committee report in 2005–2006. This committee, charged with forming policy around psychologists' "ethical" participation in interrogations, was set up by the APA to include six members (of the nine voting spots) who had current or former ties to the military establishment. According to Frank Summers (2014), a past president of Division 39, "some of (the nine) participated in the application of torture techniques at Guantanamo." Summers was calling attention to a clear conflict of interest on the part of these committee members, who were charged with formulating policy for the profession, with the apparent goal of complying with the military need to justify a legal role for psychologists in interrogations. One psychologist member resigned almost immediately in protest to the secrecy; another, Jean Maria Arrigo, who protested both the secret proceedings and the findings of the report, was vilified by a smear campaign in which the president of APA participated (Soldz, 2010).

Protest from within the APA

The earliest direct intervention by psychoanalysts as change agents was the move to withhold dues from the APA in 2006. It began with a suggestion made to the Section 9 listserv by Ghislaine Boulanger and matured into a movement beyond the Section and beyond the Division, sponsoring a website (www.ethicalapa.org) and listserv (withholddues@yahoo.org) of its own. Although several of the key figures in www.withholdapadues.org (e.g., Ruth Fallenbaum, and Ghislaine Boulanger) were and are psychoanalysts, some of the most active leaders (e.g., Dan Aalbers and Brad Olson) were not psychoanalysts. While there was controversy within the Division, psychoanalysts took the lead in grassroots activism to inform members that the APA leadership was complicit in keeping psychologists as the only health professionals participating in the abuse of prisoners. As Steven Reisner (2010) said when the issue was debated before the Council in August 2008,

> You have a rare opportunity to make a significant difference for good in the world. If I am right, and the US government believes it can only legally justify these shameful techniques by claiming medical

> supervision, then the refusal of psychologists to participate may finally put an end to these practices. At the very least, it is time you stopped psychologists from being associated with them (p. 123).

Outrage led to a petition (1 percent of the membership had to request a referendum), and after a great deal of effort and grassroots organizing, the 2008 Referendum took place, spearheaded by Dan Aalbers, Ruth Fallenbaum, and Brad Olsen, which would have prohibited psychologists from working in settings where detainees were held in violation of human rights. In psychoanalytic terms, the Referendum was an attempt to bring the unconscious (secret, hidden aspects of APA participation) into conscious awareness of the membership. It was passed by a significant majority.

But to further illustrate dissociation even among dedicated, well-meaning professionals, one of the few Council members who recognized that there were problems in ethics enforcement, Laurel Bass Wagner, asked (via email) in August 2015,

> How did no one on staff or in governance raise the question that the PENS Task Force should examine whether or not psychologists should participate in detainee interrogations and not just how to participate? How did this essential question go unasked by the APA Board of Directors?

Over the next few years, many APA members not only withheld dues, but resigned completely from the organization, as it became clear that the APA administration and the officers of other divisions were not just ignoring but opposing attempts to bring to light the role of psychologists in torture. This effort, along with other factors, has led to enough of a drop in membership that the APA has recently sent a series of letters to former members offering discounts for rejoining. Tragically, although APA leadership has repeatedly given lip service to pronouncements against torture, the principles of the Referendum have never been implemented. Discouraged by inaction and opposition, those making efforts to enforce the ethics code have been driven to work outside the structure of the APA. Some members have brought complaints—as private citizens to state boards—against some of the most egregious and public participants in the torture agenda.

Although even these efforts have not yet been successful in bringing about sanctions, they succeeded in publicizing the issue and consolidating support from APA members and former members.

Those who led the protest

What motivated the psychoanalysts who led these efforts? Ghislaine Boulanger, author of *Wounded by Reality: Understanding and Treating Adult Onset Trauma* (2007), says,

> When I learned in 2006 that the American Psychiatric Association had pulled out of Guantanamo and that the APA was only too happy to remain there, I was indignant to say the least. I did feel betrayed … knowing what I did, I felt absolute horror in imagining what was going on with these detainees, many of whom were quite young, knowing too what the psychological legacy would be. And I was privy to a number of reports (now made public) about interrogators who were developing all the symptoms of adult onset trauma, quite consistent with arguments I developed in my book. I found that being a psychoanalyst used to listening—to the extent that I could—without turning away from unbearable details, allowed me to gather information and process it in ways that were consistent with my theories about adult onset trauma.
>
> (personal communication, January 25, 2015)

Boulanger develops the point that some psychologists who participated in interrogations themselves became symptomatic of vicarious traumatization, as did some of the defense lawyers.

Laurel Bass Wagner, Division 39 member of the Council of APA, led the effort to ensure that the Council would engage in debate on this issue. Wagner, who has written about her work with the survivors of Hurricane Katrina, said that for her, psychoanalysis is "not just a two-person thing, but has always had a social responsibility component. It was important that our work not be seen as something that just occurs in the consulting room." At the same time, she feels that psychoanalytic critical listening helped her to recognize the arrogance behind the argument that psychologists are uniquely qualified to conduct interrogations or to recognize ethical "drift" in a group. She points out that psychoanalysts understand that *no* group has privileged objectivity in knowing the truth, and that these rationalizations are defensive maneuvers serving the agenda of those who wanted psychologists to participate in interrogations. "In a situation where a prisoner has no rights, there can be no informed consent. Informed consent and Do No Harm are fundamental principles of our work; in illegal detention, there is no way to not do harm." Wagner has described her own difficulty while serving as Council representative for Division 39: "It was a constant state of tension to keep from getting drawn in to the doublethink" (personal communication, January 19, 2015).

Steven Reisner (2010) writes that,

> the story we were presented with—from the Bush Administration and the American Psychological Association—about the role of psychologists and psychology in national security investigations didn't make sense … it aroused skepticism and curiosity *as a psychoanalyst*. I found myself listening *clinically* to the material … much like I listen to my patients' stories. I found myself listening for the hidden story—the story that was being obscured precisely as the surface narrative was being perfected. (p. 108)

Reisner writes further that he has realized that health professionals

> had begun to use psychological knowledge, including diagnoses and treatment, as a military tactic, even while presenting them as healing processes. I suspected a cynical misuse of diagnostic jargon, and I intuited that there was a sinister purpose embedded in the peculiarly American denial of responsibility contained in the phrase "preexisting condition." Perhaps, just as psychologists and psychiatrists on the payroll of insurance companies used this phrase to deny needed treatment, the psychologists and psychiatrists at Guantanamo were denying the effects of torture. (p. 114)

Among many other corroborating facts, Reisner's perception is validated by the APA's attempts to deny and qualify the findings of the 2004 International Commission of the Red Cross, which found that American-trained psychologists and psychiatrists were consulting on the implementation of torture at Guantanamo Bay (Soldz, 2010).

Duties to members, or duties of members?

Has a national organization harmed its members by secretly acting to forge ties with senior CIA and Pentagon officials and by failing to effectively enforce its own ethics code? In commenting on the Risen book and on the recent release of the Senate Select Committee Report on Intelligence, which both reveal new information on the role of psychologists in detention settings, Frank Summers (2014) wrote in an email to Division 39, "[W]e now have new clarity on the APA agenda. It has been working hand in glove with the Pentagon and the CIA while adopting a policy of benign neglect to the wishes of its own members."

The conditions of institutional betrayal described by Smith and Freyd have apparently been fulfilled; the APA as an institution has clearly harmed its members through deception, betrayal, and subversion of the ethics code. Care for the inner well-being of clients is at the very core of this profession, which values the integrity of subjective experience. Lies and double messages have harmed psychoanalysts, psychologists, and those who seek their services, both now and in the future.

In her landmark book *Trauma and Recovery*, Judith Herman (1996) said that the final stage in recovery from trauma is reconnection with community. So it is not surprising that many of the psychoanalysts drawn to oppose the APA's inaction on torture were themselves trauma therapists, who understood the impact and importance of torture both on an individual and systems level, and who were also strongly drawn to create a community of like-minded psychoanalysts who shared the deep compassionate identification with torture victims and could help heal themselves in the community of concerned fellow analysts. We as psychoanalysts and psychologists needed and still need to heal ourselves and our community from the institutional betrayal of the secrecy and collusion that poisoned the organization we had come to rely on and identify with.

One of the most important lessons we could learn from these events is how very hard it is to recognize and come to accept that institutional betrayal has taken place. The essential information in the Hoffman report—that the APA administration was saying one thing and doing the exact opposite—was fully available on the websites mentioned above for more than a decade and repeatedly and consistently raised in professional contexts (Soldz, 2010). The Referendum passed in 2008 prohibiting participation in interrogations and directing APA leadership to enforce this policy was not implemented by investigations and sanctions until a change in the Ethics code was recently (2016) opened for comments. This inaction was despite Laurel Bass Wagner's assertion in an email to Division 56 (Trauma) that "Division 39 asked every president in the seven years (following) to implement it, to no avail." More members voted in the Referendum than generally vote in the yearly election of officers, yet none of the well-documented ethics charges brought against current or former members ever resulted in any enforcement. Rather, these complaints were met with excessive demands for further documentation, silence, delays, and/or aggression against those bringing the complaints.

Kenneth Pope (2015), former ethics director of APA, raises the importance of the role of the "bystander," members who supported the APA by paying dues and sharing in whatever benefits derived from membership. Pope, like Zimbardo, suggests that we each search our souls in the light of what we now know about human behavior in groups and about individual denial of responsibility, and examine our participation in society

> carefully before we judge or blame others rather than ourselves. As we go about taking steps to make ethics stronger in organizations, this study reminds us that a chance to make a difference can come at an inconvenient time and catch us off guard by appearing in forms we did not expect, that we can pass by it without noticing, and that we need to pay attention to what shows up unannounced at every step.
>
> (2015, p. 150)

No doubt there is a duty of membership, as there is a duty of officership. But where access to procedural knowledge is restricted or made hard to get, members will be discouraged. And above all, there is the pull to dissociate from knowledge that contradicts existing power structures and conventional arrangements, as discussed below.

Thus, the militarization of American society has come to be accepted, as more than half of all taxes go to "defense," and the "enhanced interrogation" of the Bush Administration became a norm through the "ticking bomb scenario," the dramatic distortion of a fictional need for torture to save lives. This misleading scenario, along with the false ideas that torture can produce reliable intelligence information and emergencies justify impulsive action, has invaded public perception of "terrorists" through popular TV shows like "*24*." An example of the misuse of the "emergency" claim by the APA Board of Directors might be the 2005 declaration of an emergency, bypassing the normal review by Council, which would have allowed for evaluation and debate about approval of the PENS report. The APA then repeatedly and falsely claimed that the Council had endorsed the report. The report then stood as policy until 2013, despite objections and token corrections to the official record. In order to fully understand why the membership did not object more strongly to what was clearly wrong in retrospect, we would need to fully accept the reality of social construction of the social unconscious and its power to confuse and obscure whatever challenges existing power arrangements. We also need to grasp the power of media manipulation and disinformation strategies, as in this example, and the importance of thorough public discussion of an organization's ethics policies.

Given the importance of the unconscious social construction in shaping personal values and attitudes, how could the writers of any ethics code be expected to completely transcend their own bias, and even more simply, their own self-interest? Ethicist Laura Stark (2015) has written:

> The elite professionals who are empowered to write and change an ethics policy have tremendous influence over its content. But ethics policies are anonymous because they have force only to the extent that they appear to represent the position of an entire organization, not a few powerful people. The process is designed to erase the mark of those heavy hands who wrote the rules for everybody.

Stark recommends that we "give the code of ethics a byline" in order to aid recognition of bias. Kenneth Pope (2015), a former ethics director of the APA, has written a comprehensive review of barriers to organizational ethics enforcement, and Reisner and Soldz (Risen, 2015 and emails to Division 39) have also put forward concise and specific steps needed immediately to redress the harm.

But an important structural problem may also contribute to issues of ethics enforcement. Like most professional associations, APA administration and governance are made up of two very different groups: salaried permanent staff, and part-time volunteers elected by Divisions through votes by membership. The terms of service of the elected volunteers are more temporary, often as little as a year of president-elect followed by a year of service as president of a division and a third year as past president. Institutional power and memory thus gravitate to the more permanent, full-time personnel, who have tactical power in terms of access to officials, relationships, and funds that have to be collected and cultivated over time. Elected officers often turn to "permanent" staff for information about procedures. Due to the temporary terms of office of these elected officers, they are dependent on the administrators for access to resources of all kinds, including interpretations of procedures and policies. This mixed governance structure has the potential in all professional organizations to lead to institutional splits in which the administrators use their inherent power to serve other needs than those of the membership. The guild model of professions has changed over time due to the need for permanent salaried employees who now carry and control the institutional memory. The economic basis of the organization plays a part, too—membership dues make up only a small part of the yearly income of the APA; a major portion of that income comes from real estate and other investments, which limit the financial influence members can have. In sum, any effective review of ethics problems in APA must consider the social, organizational, and structural barriers to ethics enforcement as well as the unconscious motivations.

Much can be learned from this prolonged sad and shocking episode about organizations, membership participation (or lack of it), personal and institutional integrity, and ethics enforcement (or lack of it). Let us hope that we can take in all the painful truth that will strengthen us as members and professionals to become more active and vigilant with and for those who represent us, and more aware and accepting of the public and community duties of professional life.

References

Boulanger, G. (2007). *Wounded by Reality: Understanding and Treating Adult Onset Trauma*. New York: Routledge.

Feinstein, D. (2014). Senate intelligence study on CIA detention and interrogation program. Retrieved from www.feinstein.senate.gov/public/index.cfm/senate-intelligence-committee-study-on-cia-detention-and-interrogation-program, accessed January 17, 2016.

Harris, A., and Botticelli, S. (2010). *First Do No Harm: The Paradoxical Encounters of Psychoanalysis, Warmaking, and Resistance*. New York: Routledge.

Herman, J. L. (1996). *Trauma and Recovery: The Aftermath of Violence—From Domestic Abuse to Political Terror*. New York: Basic Books.

Hoffman, D. H. (2015). Report to the special committee of the board of directors of the American Psychological Association: Independent review relating to

APA guidelines, national security interrogations, and torture. Retrieved from www.apa.org/independent-review/APA-FINAL-Report-7.2.15.pdf, accessed January 2, 2016.

Hollander, N. (January 2014). What's in the frame? Clinical challenges in a time of social malaise. Paper presented to the Psychoanalytic Institute of Northern California, San Francisco, CA.

Milgram, S. (1983). *Obedience to Authority*. New York: Harper Perennial.

Pope, K. S. (2015). Steps to strengthen ethics in organizations: Research findings, ethics placebos, and what works. *Journal of Trauma and Dissociation, 16*(2), 139–152.

Pope, K. S. (2016). The Hoffman report and the American Psychological Association: Meeting the challenge of change. In K. S. Pope and M. J. T. Vasquez (Eds), *Ethics in Psychotherapy and Counseling: A Practical Guide* (5th edition.) (pp. 361–369). Hoboken: John Wiley and Sons.

Reisner, S. (2010). From resistance to resistance: A narrative of psychoanalytic activism. In A. Harris and S. Botticelli (Eds), *First Do No Harm: The Paradoxical Encounters of Psychoanalysis, Warmaking, and Resistance* (pp. 107–141). New York: Routledge.

Risen, J. (2014). *Pay any Price: Greed, Power and Endless War*. New York: Houghton Mifflin Harcourt.

Risen, J. (2015). All the president's psychologists: APA's secret complicity with government in support of CIA torture program. Retrieved from http://leaksource.info/2015/05/08/all-the-presidents-psychologists-apa-secret-complicity-with-govt-in-support-of-cia-torture-program/, accessed December 15, 2015.

Smith, C. P., and Freyd, J. J. (2014). Institutional betrayal. *American Psychologist, 69*(6), 575–587.

Soldz, S. (2010). Psychologists defying torture: The challenge and the path ahead. In A. Harris and S. Botticelli (Eds), *First Do No Harm: The Paradoxical Encounters of Psychoanalysis, Warmaking, and Resistance* (pp. 67–105). New York: Routledge.

Stark, L. (July 21, 2015). Why ethics codes fail. Retrieved from www.insidehighered.com/views/2015/07/21/essay-why-scholarly-ethics-codes-may-be-likely-fail, accessed August 13, 2015.

Summers, Frank, Ph.D., ABPP. (December 19, 2014). President of Division 39 (Psychoanalysis) "Psychologists' Involvement in Torture and the APA" by Kristi Pikiewicz, Ph.D., in *Meaningful You*, a blog that curates the voices of Division 39.

Vasquez, M. J. T. (2016). Appendix B: The Hoffman report: Resetting APA's moral compass. In K. S. Pope and M. J. T. Vasquez (Eds), *Ethics in Psychotherapy and Counseling: A Practical Guide* (5th edition) (pp. 370–379). Hoboken: John Wiley and Sons.

Zimbardo, P. (2008). *The Lucifer Effect: Understanding How Good People Turn Evil*. New York: Random House.

Chapter 13

Robert Jay Lifton

A witness and prophet who feels deeply and assaults our minds[1]

Lewis Aron

It was an enormous honor for me to welcome Robert Jay Lifton to New York University where he presented a paper entitled "Witness to an Extreme Century: Thoughts on Scholarship and Activism" and I remain grateful for the privilege of being asked to comment on his presentation and on his extraordinary memoir *Witness to an Extreme Century*. Thanks to the enthusiastic scholarship of Judie Alpert and Liz Goren I am now able to add some additional reflections on their probing interview "The Analyst as Witness, Historian and Activist: A Conversation with Robert Jay Lifton" with particular reference to the two topics mentioned in the title of Dr. Lifton's paper—scholarship and social activism—but here more specifically focusing on psychoanalytic education and social activism, two areas that are intricately, but problematically, related.

Lifton speaks as a wise, deeply engaged, and ethically charged, indeed prophetic, witness to an extreme century. Prophets, we know, are not those who predict the future but are constituted by their impassioned plea for morality and justice. Abraham Heschel (1962) described prophets as those who "feel fiercely" (p. 5), "assault our minds" (p. 12), and challenge our sacred certainties and institutions, exposing our scandalous pretensions. In his article Lifton mentions that when he was contemplating his work with Nazi doctors, several Jewish friends advised him that Judiasm advocated that we "let evil lie." But all one needs to do is read Heschel's study of the prophets to counter that misleading claim. The prophet, however, bears scorn and reproach, and witnessing is dangerous; witnesses risk being killed for their testimonies, hence martyrdom derives from bearing witness and it is just this danger that makes witnessing sacred. In the words of Amos 5:10:

> They hate him who reproves in the gate,
> They abhor him who speaks the truth.

Of the many topics addressed by Lifton, his thoughts on scholarship and activism are perhaps the most significant for me to address in my role as the director of New York University's (NYU) Postdoctoral Program in Psychotherapy and Psychoanalysis. In his memoir and in the interview, Lifton describes his own troubled and still evolving relationship with psychoanalysis, to which he has always been drawn, and is yet wary of embracing because of his "allergy to totalism." For a time early in his career he pursued psychoanalytic training, being analyzed by the Freudian, Beate Rank, former wife of Otto, a woman Freud described as like a daughter to him, and he was deeply influenced by psychoanalysts of a variety of orientations, classical, interpersonal, and idiosyncratic, particularly his mentor and friend, Erik Erikson. He distanced himself from the "totalism" of psychoanalytic institutes and from the rigidities of its orthodoxy. I want to highlight aspects of the psycho-history of psychoanalysis regarding scholarship and activism, the micro and the macro, the individual and the socio-political, the scholar–clinician and "the psychoanalyst citizen" (Gourguechon, 2011).

In its European origins psychoanalysis was a progressive movement, with many of the analysts leftists, and at the very least liberals, if not outright communists. It was a movement that began exclusively, and then predominantly, among newly emancipated Jews who were immigrants and the children of immigrants, who had often fled poverty and persecution, and who now sublimated their Jewish particularistic values into universalistic ethical and culturally Greek/German Enlightenment attitudes. Like Marxism with which it was so often compared and connected, it had strong elements of universal Messianic aspirations. Karen Starr and I took the title of our recent book, *A Psychotherapy for the People*, directly from Freud who in 1918 charged psychoanalysts with making psychoanalysis available to the uneducated and the poor. Psychoanalysts were socially active, as Danto (2005) has meticulously documented, in establishing "free clinics," in developing early childhood education, in providing sex education and birth control to young adults, and participated directly in liberal and radical political causes. It is also true, however, that Freud was wary of too direct a connection between the psychoanalytic movement and politics out of fear of anti-Semitism, that too much activism would harm psychoanalysis. We know that the Nazis did in fact lump together and outlaw Freudian psychoanalysis, Marxism, Einsteinian physics with its relativity, and Boasian anthropology with its politically active critique of racial categorization, as "Jewish sciences."

As the émigrés fled Hitler and following the Second World War as America became the center of the psychoanalytic world in its golden years, two trends joined together to de-radicalize psychoanalysis. The first factor was the medicalization of American psychoanalysis, and the second was the de-radicalization of the émigrés as they adapted to a new home following trauma.

Against Freud's wishes, psychoanalysis in America joined itself with medicine and psychiatry. Psychoanalysis played a part throughout the twentieth century in transforming psychiatry from a poorly regarded, low-status, administrative, and caretaking asylum-based occupation to a high-status and lucrative private practice medical specialty. Freud came to America just at the time that the Flexner report began the process of the professionalization of medicine and the accreditation of medical education. Psychoanalysis would align itself with psychiatry and professional medicine following the polarization of care and treatment. Care is what was provided to the incurable, to those who could not be treated. Care is what doctors had done before medicine became scientific, but now psychoanalysis, like medicine, left care to others and wanted to provide and be associated with treatment. Treatment was carried out by doctors, the largely male medical profession. Psychoanalysis embraced the values of treatment, and care was projected outward, assigned to the necessary and yet devalued "supportive" psychotherapy, often carried out by the social worker wives of the analysts.

Whereas professional medicine, with its entrepreneurial spirit, was a male, men's business—in the 1950s over 90 percent of analysts were men and this number was increasing in private practice—social activism and reform movements were associated with masculine, moralizing women; the abolitionists and prohibitionists were key examples of this. In America, reformers and social workers were mainly women who were paid little and devalued (Danto, 2009). The psychoanalyst émigrés, who had just lost so much, and who wanted to fit in and adapt to their new home, one that had saved their lives, joined together with a younger generation of American doctors who sought to establish psychoanalysis as pure and medical—a scientific treatment, a prestigious profession. Those who were not medical doctors, and not welcome within the American psychoanalytic mainstream, often took agency positions here and joined with what Freud had called the salvation army of social workers. Prior to emigrating from Austria to the United States when the Nazis rose to power, Otto Fenichel wrote from a socialist perspective, and then once in the United States he wrote almost exclusively about clinical matters (Jacoby, 1983). He worked himself to death, dying while trying to obtain a medical license. Generally, as their focus becomes more narrowly clinical, clinicians become more socially conservative (Kupers, 2009). Jewish émigrés fled an anti-Semitic Europe in which Jewish men were thought to be effeminate, perverse, and homosexual, and so they were happy to be welcomed in America as psychoanalysts at a time that it was a male, medical, scientific profession, held in high esteem, and embracing stereotypically masculine sensibilities that emphasized independence and ego-autonomy. Hence, what happened to psychoanalysis in America was the result of a perfect storm of racism, anti-Semitism, misogyny, and homophobia.

Under these circumstances, psychoanalysis aligned itself with science, purity, professionalization, and medical treatment, and split itself off from supportive care, social work, nursing, and political activism, all that was categorized as effeminate, and at best, denigrated as "applied." The mid-century psychoanalytic leader Lawrence Kubie, who himself did a great deal to rescue the émigrés, forcefully argued that psychoanalysts should not engage in the public sphere because they should be immersed in clinical practice, preserve their anonymity, and stick to what they know, namely, the inner world of their individual patients (Gourgeuchon, 2011). While there were voices to the contrary, and while as individuals many analysts were socially active and even radical, psychoanalysis as a movement and as a profession took the more cautious and conservative path.

Much has changed in psychoanalysis. In a recent plenary address to the American Psychoanalytic Association, former president Prudence Gourguechon (2011) made a strong case of "the citizen psychoanalyst" and under my own presidency, Division 39 created a Section of psychoanalysts for social responsibility. Psychoanalytic education, as Lifton acknowledges, is now more open, democratic, and pluralistic. We have made substantial progress, as psychoanalysis has increasingly become a women's profession, and of lesser status than in its golden years, on such matters as misogyny, homophobia, and racism. But we have a long way to go. Even now, and even in New York City, how much attention is being paid in psychoanalytic institutes to such practical matters as poverty, homelessness, immigration, the devastation of the union movement, nuclear threat, and political oppression? There are notable exceptions: Neil Altman (2010) stands out as among the singular voices for his work on psychoanalysis in the inner city; Nancy Hollander's (2010) social psychoanalysis of terrorism in the Americas; Sue Grand (2013), with her call for a psychoanalysis addressing social justice. Increasingly we hear these calls for the revitalization of psychoanalysis, challenging the disengaged. Taking up such matters is too often pathologized, thought to reflect grandiosity and omnipotence, while neglecting such topics remains normative. How many of us even consider interpreting to our patients along the lines suggested by Kupers (2009, p. 583): "Why are you choosing to come see me for therapy and Prozac instead of joining in solidarity with your fellow workers to wrest control of the workplace from the managers?" I, however, would want to modify this question so as to clarify that the patient might do both rather than either/or.

The interview makes clear that there is an enormous distinction between psychoanalysis as an intellectual set of ideas and psychoanalysis as a movement, profession, and guild. As Dr. Lifton makes clear, psychoanalytic ideas have consistently sparked the interest of brilliant and creative thinkers across disciplines, even while psychoanalytic institutions were conservative, doctrinaire, and rigid. As he also points out, this is directly tied to the theme of intergenerational transmission as so many generations of psychoanalysts inherited the "trauma" of rigidified forms of psychoanalytic education. Among the many ideas that caught my attention was Dr. Lifton's tongue in cheek comment that "There was something useful about confronting the prevailing orthodoxy of the time, in order to deepen one's own heresy." I do think that many of the outstanding newer ideas in psychoanalysis evolved as counter-reactions to established doctrines that cried out for challenge. Some of these ideas were later reincorporated into psychoanalysis, without their originator necessarily receiving due credit, but others have remained marginal altogether. I would add that the conservative stance of institutes was directly tied to the homogeneity of psychoanalysis during its "halcyon years." Psychoanalysis was disproportionately male, White, Jewish, upwardly mobile middle-class, and heterosexual. This homogeneity, and particularly the related guild mentality of protecting shared financial interests, contributed to the conservativism of institutes. In our day and age, and for the future survival of psychoanalysis, we need a dual focus on both the application of psychoanalysis to the wider world, to social activism, and to diversity. These go together because so many professionals who are potentially interested in psychoanalysis come from ethnic, religious, and class groups that are underrepresented within the psychoanalytic profession and it is often these very people who are in the best position to bring psychoanalysis back to their communities, if and only if psychoanalysis can change and grow such that it is applicable to situations outside of the "private practice" economy. There is a serious question to be considered about whether we want to lose potential candidates like Dr. Lifton by maintaining our narrow rigidities or whether we can genuinely open psychoanalysis up to be used in new ways, in novel settings, among people who until now would not have seen themselves as potential beneficiaries of psychoanalysis. Can the very definition of psychoanalysis grow, expand, and transform while remaining true to its core basis? And can the profession diversify in all kinds of ways so that we are more like the world that we want to understand and treat?

Lifton begins his memoir by attributing his own social activism to his identification with the victims. After what he had witnessed it became urgent for him to speak out against mind-control, nuclear weapons, American war-making, and Nazi-like cruelty and genocide. Dr. Lifton wonders about how much his Jewish background impacted his attitudes and scholarship, but much of religion is rooted in the theme that we learn empathy through our identification with suffering, whether we meditate on the passion of Christ or experience ourselves being freed from slavery to Pharaoh. When in the 1970s at Yale (I was there for this event, by the way), Lifton explained to Jacques Lacan that symbolization could replace the centrality of drives in psychoanalytic theory, Lacan responded "Je suis Liftonian!" (Lifton, 2011, p. 367). I think today many analysts would agree with Lifton's arguments, but particularly with his call for our ongoing engagement in both scholarship and activism. In my plea for a progressive psychoanalysis, a psychotherapy for the people, I too call on all of us to be Liftonion!

Note

1 This chapter was initially presented as an introduction to a colloquium held at New York University on April 4, 2012, co-sponsored by the NYU Interdisciplinary Freud Research Group and the NYU-GSAS Trauma and Violence Transdisciplinary Studies Program. My thanks to the Interdisciplinary Freud Research Group and the NYU-GSAS Trauma and Violence Transdisciplinary Studies Program and especially to Judie Alpert and Liz Goren for inviting me to participate both in that symposium and in this collection. I have rewritten the chapter incorporating some reflections on their interview of Dr. Lifton.

References

Altman, N. (2010). *The Analyst in the Inner City, Second Edition.* NY: Routledge.

Aron, L. and Starr, K. (2013). *A Psychotherapy for the People.* London and NY: Routledge.

Danto, E. A. (2005). *Freud's Free Clinics.* NY: Columbia University Press.

Danto, E. A. (2009). A new sort of 'Salvation Army': Historical perspectives on the confluence of psychoanalysis and social work. *Clinical Social Work,* 37: 67–76.

Gourguechon, P. L. (2011). The citizen psychoanalyst: Psychoanalysis, social commentary, and social advocacy. *Journal of the American Psychoanalytic Association,* 59: 445–470.

Grand, S. (2013). God at an impasse: Devotion, social justice, and the psychoanalytic subject. *Psychoanalytical Dialogues,* 23: 449–463.

Heschel, A. (1962). *The Prophets.* NY: Harper and Row Publishers.

Hollander, N. C. (2010). *Uprooted Minds.* NY: Routledge.

Jacoby, R. (1983). *The Repression of Psychoanalysis.* NY: Basic Books.

Kupers, T. A. (2009). The turn away from social activism in psychoanalysis. *Journal of the American Academy of Psychoanalysis and Dynamic Psychiatry,* 37: 581–586.

Lifton, R. J. (2011). *Witness to an Extreme Century: A Memoir.* NY: Free Press.

Conclusion

Psychoanalysis, trauma, and community: Lessons learned

Alison Lake, Elizabeth R. Goren, and Judith L. Alpert

As reviewed both in the introduction to this volume and in the chapter by Lewis Aron, psychoanalysis has a long history of progressive social engagement, which fell into abeyance during the period following World War II. Despite the now indelible image of the psychoanalyst sequestered in a well-appointed office uncovering the intrapsychic conflicts of one paying patient at a time, a new trend is emerging that sees contemporary psychoanalysts reengaging with social issues and—once again—offering therapeutic services to a broader spectrum of the world's population. The contributors to this volume offer examples of the kinds of work psychoanalysts can do when they apply their expertise outside the traditional treatment room.

It is no accident that a book about therapeutic interventions in community settings is also a book about trauma. The enclosed space of the treatment room and an inward focus on early childhood experiences and intrapsychic issues are suited to one another. With the opening of the office door, passages can be made in two directions: an accounting for socio-political and other environmental causes of human suffering can enter into the treatment, while the analyst can exit the office to meet suffering individuals in the contexts where they live. The chapters in this book show us analysts at work with runaways in train stations, with displaced people in Red Cross shelters, with workers in occupied factories, with residents in racially segregated towns, and with enemy groups in geographic regions characterized by longstanding ethnic and national conflict. The work performed in these diverse settings reflects the analysts' engagement with the traumatic impacts of such forces as generational poverty and racial discrimination, war and other forms of political violence, and massive natural disasters.

What kinds of interventions can psychoanalysts offer to mitigate the psychic impacts of trauma when they leave traditional treatment settings behind? This concluding chapter will review four general approaches taken by contributors to this volume to working with and in traumatized communities. It will end by suggesting ways psychoanalysts and psychoanalytic institutes might support the flourishing of this kind of work.

Receiving testimony

Brushes with death and other profound insults to self can leave trauma survivors with memories that defy symbolization, and therefore with losses that cannot be effectively mourned. The difficulty experienced by survivors in representing and communicating their experiences, moreover, can leave these experiences veiled in silence, and unshared. Dori Laub (this volume, Chapter 1) relates the failure of symbolization of experiences of terror to the destruction of the empathic internalized object that makes dialogue, and thought itself, possible. In order to reverse this process, he makes himself available as an attuned, empathic listener to receive the testimonies of Holocaust survivors. As a listener prepared in advance to tolerate and absorb the intense affects associated with traumatic memories, Laub joins the survivor in retracing the story of his or her life from childhood to the present, without omitting the intervening traumatic episodes that may previously have gone unowned and undescribed. As the survivor's story is heard by the trained, empathic listener, the survivor's internal good object begins to be restored, and the survivor comes to hear and to know his or her own story as well, in a way that had not previously been possible. The effects of this restoration of dialogue are manifold. As Laub describes, memories once symbolized can be not only shared, reducing the isolation and loneliness of the survivor, but also forgotten, leaving the survivor more free to live in the present. Once recorded and archived, moreover, the testimonies received can be made available to wider audiences, facilitating a broader, social acknowledgment of these "lived realities" that may be key to healing not only the survivors themselves, but society at large (see Ainslie, this volume).

Judy Roth (this volume, Chapter 2) offers herself as empathic "companion–listener" (in Laub's words) to individuals whose traumatic exposure is not past but ongoing. In traveling to speak with those living in zones of ongoing political violence, Roth describes the potential benefits to traumatized individuals of having their experiences of brutality and uncertainty validated and contained by a psychoanalytically informed witness, even in the midst of ongoing danger. She openly questions whether her "accompaniment" may not pose risks as well, insofar as her support may awaken hopes that are not realistic, or may enable traumatized individuals to relax defenses such as denial, disavowal, and minimization which are in fact crucial to their ongoing psychic survival in a conflict zone. Overarching this dilemma is Roth's concern with the wider social and political effects of our collective denial of violence and suffering. As an advocate for those who have shared their stories with her, she seeks to "amplify" their voices and to spread awareness of their experiences, thereby mitigating against the widespread wish, on the part of those outside the conflict zones, not to see, hear, or know about terror. At this collective level, too, she seeks to make the unknowable known. Finally, Roth writes of the ways her contacts with victims of political violence in the Middle East change her as a therapist, enabling her better to see the effects of socio-political forces such as racism and prejudice on those she meets in her New York City office.

Therapeutic encounters outside the frame

Disasters, whether natural or man-made, disrupt survivors' lives and livelihoods and can compromise their abilities to trust others and to trust the world as a safe place. Many people in need of therapeutic intervention after such crises are thus unlikely to seek office-based mental health treatment. Psychoanalysts have been led out of their comfort zones and familiar territories by the desire to help these survivors (see, e.g., Levy et al., 2004), and the interventions offered outside the traditional office setting have necessarily differed from those offered within it. Goren (2011) has described her psychoanalytic engagement with firefighters, conducted onsite in firehouses in New York City after 9/11, as a kind of "therapy on the run." She interacted with firefighters on their own turf, on a catch-as-catch-can basis, because that was the only way to access this group of people in need of healing but unwilling (at least at first) to participate in more traditional, scheduled treatment. The related experiences of contributors to this volume help us to ask and begin to answer questions like the following: What is psychoanalysis without the crucial element of the psychoanalytic frame? What defines an interaction as psychoanalytic when it takes place outside the office, outside the regularly scheduled 50-minute hour, outside an ongoing treatment relationship, without the ability either to withhold or to carefully titrate personal information about the therapist, or without stable and mutually established agreements regarding each party's role?

Laurel Bass Wagner (this volume, Chapter 3) writes of bringing a psychoanalytic perspective to disaster response, the acute phase of work with trauma victims in the immediate aftermath of a traumatic event. The displaced survivors of Hurricane Katrina, with whom Wagner worked, experienced broken attachments, broken trust, extreme resource loss, and myriad other insults to self. Faced with a sea of displaced people in the Dallas Red Cross shelters, Wagner soon learned that it was infeasible to offer treatment on an individual basis. Despite this, she maintained a commitment to getting to know the survivors and a sensitivity to eliciting their particular needs. For example, she was able to identify displaced children's needs for transitional objects, and to recognize something as mundane as racially appropriate hair care products, requested by survivors who had begun to feel seen by her, as a real psychological resource, capable of supporting both a restoration of lost dignity and a reconnection with normal human experience. In her recalled conversations with survivors in the shelters, drawing on the principles of psychological first aid, Wagner reflects on survivors' strength and resiliency in order to shore up their damaged senses of themselves as valuable and competent, and offers resources and reassurances to help restore lost feelings of safety and normalcy. Whereas psychological first aid generally recommends against the survivor's exploring feelings and talking about the traumatic experience in its immediate aftermath, Wagner's understanding that traumatic impacts differ depending upon preexisting levels of psychological functioning and on the cumulative effects of past trauma, enabled her to recommend a more flexible stance, grounded in attunement to individuals who may or may not be ready and eager to tell their stories. Across the varied interactions she describes, Wagner's chapter testifies to the value of her attending to the current relationship between herself and her interlocutors for clues to their most pressing anxieties and needs.

Ghislaine Boulanger (this volume, Chapter 4) describes the experiences of psychoanalysts working in New Orleans at the time of Hurricane Katrina, who continued to offer services to their patients even as they themselves experienced displacement and other impacts of trauma. Even those who did not leave their offices, or who attempted to maintain the traditional analytic frame, found that frame disrupted. They found themselves impelled into makeshift offices, new schedules, and a new transparency about their own circumstances in relation to the disaster. Analysts and patients alike experienced the needs to have their resilience supported and normalcy restored. As analysts worked in parallel with their patients to symbolize and assimilate what had happened to them, some of the traditional asymmetry in the analytic relationship was lost, and boundaries and roles at times became blurred. Boulanger describes how this destabilization of the analytic frame could leave analysts feeling vulnerable and deskilled, but also, in the best-case outcomes, appreciative of a new basis for empathy with their patients.

Neil Altman (this volume, Chapter 5) is drawn to engage in therapy "out of the office" or "on the run" not in response to a disaster but by the desire to make psychoanalysis available to suffering people in lower socio-economic classes and in the developing world, for whom office-based treatment may be not only inaccessible but also culturally alien. He describes therapeutic interventions that take place in chaotic environments and during spontaneous, chance encounters with individuals subject to chronically traumatic conditions such as extreme poverty. What makes these encounters psychoanalytic, for Altman, is the attention paid to unconscious process, to transference and countertransference dynamics as they emerge even without the projection of an analytic blank screen, and to the flow of feelings and anxieties (both one's own and one's interlocutor's) over the course of the interaction. Altman seeks in these encounters to offer comments that show people that they have been heard, and that help them to mentalize their own almost unthinkable emotional experiences; he holds that psychoanalytic work such as this can be done anywhere. Just as for the traumatized analysts Boulanger describes, the abilities to attend to and to tolerate one's own emotional reactions are key for analysts and other mental health practitioners working via spontaneous interactions in traumatized communities.

Facilitating collective mourning

Survivors of trauma can experience a profound sense of isolation, and a sense of removal from ordinary human experience with no felt possibility of return. In the words of Doris Brothers, following Kohut, "it is only by regaining a sense of being 'a human among humans' ... that we have any hope of emerging from the unbearably lonely exile of trauma" (Brothers, 2009, p. 56). Although, as we have seen, this return to feeling once again "human among humans" can be catalyzed by an encounter with a single, attuned listener, recognition of one's own experience in the experience of other survivors can also have a powerful effect. "Because traumatized people feel so alienated by their experience, survivor groups have a special place in the recovery process" (Herman, 1992, p. 215). When trauma has impacted an entire community, moreover, the most effective interventions may take place at the community level. Collectively experienced losses may necessitate the initiation of collective mourning processes in order for healing to be achieved, and to endure. Finally, the "survivor mission" (Herman, 1992; see also Lifton, this volume, Chapter 9) which helps repair a survivor's senses of agency, control, and meaning can also take a collective form, such as in movements for reparative social change. What might it look like for psychoanalysts to facilitate these modes of collective healing? Three contributors to this volume provide examples of analysts engaged in group-directed trauma interventions.

Ricardo Ainslie (this volume, Chapter 6) writes of a set of three interventions developed for a Texas town traumatized by a long and ongoing history of racial discrimination. Like Wagner in the Red Cross shelters, he approached the situation by making efforts to get to know members of the community and in the process learning from them their most salient emotional needs. He and his team found many Black residents eager to speak about a piece of their shared history—the closing and razing of a historically Black school—that had suffered public erasure. Ainslie's first intervention was therefore, like Laub, to provide a forum where traumatized individuals, in conversation with trained listeners, could offer their testimony (or *testimonio*, in the Latin American tradition) about this intensely felt event. The second intervention was to create from the recordings of these testimonies a documentary film, and to screen it, facilitating a wider, public recognition of the erased events and of their lasting emotional impact. The third intervention was the organization of a public event that constituted, in Ainslie's conception, a psychoanalytic interpretation of the unspoken conflicts underlying contemporary race relations in the town. This memorial event was designed both to acknowledge feelings of loss, and to celebrate the value the school had had to many; it was designed to bring together both Black and White participants; and it included the establishment of a permanent memorial display. These interventions enabled people who may have felt alone with painful memories, and isolated by anger and resentment, to connect, first with one listener, next with others who shared similar experiences, and finally with those on the other side of their town's racial divide. Taken together, they provided platforms for a traumatized community to verbalize its experiences, to have them acknowledged, and to take reparative action, thus bringing the past into explicit and constructive engagement with the present.

In her chapter, Donna Bassin (this volume, Chapter 7) describes the years-long journey which brought her from an initial curiosity about post-9/11 veterans' movements, to the design of a large-scale art installation, developed to support community grieving for military personnel killed both in action and by suicide. Finding combat veterans engaged in creative acts of "self-witnessing," she felt compelled as a psychoanalyst not to join the general public's "violence of silence" (Chapter 7) regarding the consequences of war, but instead to create expanded opportunities for non-veterans to join in this witnessing. Her first intervention took the form of a documentary film, designed, like Ainslie's, to provide a public platform for testimonial voices. Bassin further saw veterans grappling with ongoing needs to name and to mourn both their losses and their moral injuries, but lacking a safe, containing space in which to do so. She offered her informed support to Combat Paper NJ, recognizing the therapeutic value in creative interventions that allowed veterans to metabolize traumatic experiences in the company of other veterans, using not only verbal but also artistic self-expression. She envisions the upcoming warehouse-sized installation of Combat Paper artwork as offering, both concretely and symbolically, a safe, containing space where veterans and civilians can come together to share accountability, and to bear witness.

Vamik Volkan (this volume, Chapter 8) brings psychoanalytic insight to bear on psychopolitical problems on perhaps the largest scale of any of our contributors. The "Tree Model" described in his chapter aims to address the sequelae of traumatic experiences of victimization that impact not only whole societies, but multiple generations. He describes how members of nations, ethnic groups, and other large social groups come to embrace memories of particular traumatic events as timelessly central to their identities, as well as how both this identification and the unresolved psychological tasks it entails are transmitted from one generation to the next. Under these circumstances, "tens, hundreds of thousands, or millions of people" can be trapped in a common "inability to mourn" (Chapter 8).

Meanwhile, resentment against the perceived victimizer remains intransigent. Volkan is careful to note that memorials to such losses can have the effects either of facilitating mourning, or of celebrating resentment and marking the refusal to mourn. The intervention he describes involves: (1) a series of psychoanalytically informed interviews with members of the opposing large groups, which provide necessary education to the intervention's facilitators; (2) a series of psychopolitical dialogues (which may span years) between members of the opposing groups, moderated by psychoanalytically informed facilitators sensitive to large-group identity issues; and finally, (3) the enactment of policies, laws, and other concrete changes which publicize and operationalize the insights gained. Through these stages, key conscious and unconscious conflicts are identified, historical grievances are aired, psychological obstacles to reconciliation are uncovered and addressed, and a project for social change is adopted at the large-group level. By the end, it should be possible for the large group's "chosen trauma"—like the once-frozen traumatic memories of Laub's individual survivors—to belong finally to the past.

Psychoanalytic scholarship and activism

One of the forces that can contribute to the emotional isolation of trauma survivors is a tendency on the part of the general public—psychoanalysts included—to want not to know about terror (see Roth, Chapter 2, and see also Lifton, Chapter 9). Psychoanalysts functioning as scholars and as activists have the capacity to counteract this tendency by bringing traumatic events, traumatogenic social conditions, and their sequelae into public awareness. However, as noted by Nina Thomas in her Foreword and by Judy Roth in Chapter 2, denial can at times be necessary to mental health. The safety of a holding environment may then be needed in order for acknowledgment of our own or others' lived realities (see Ainslie, Chapter 6) to be both feasible and constructive. A psychoanalytic office—and more importantly, a psychoanalytic relationship—can provide this containment. Our contributors thus far have demonstrated diverse methods for creating such safe relational spaces outside of clinical offices. This next section extends the possibility that a sensitively applied psychoanalytic understanding can—in writing, teaching, or other extra-therapeutic social engagement—itself provide a framework within which uncomfortable realities can be constructively addressed.

Although Robert Jay Lifton, interviewed by Elizabeth Goren and Judie Alpert (this volume, Chapter 9), may no longer identify as a psychoanalyst, he participates in the intellectual history of psychoanalysis and in the project of bringing psychoanalysis into history. He perceives it as imperative for the psychoanalyst or psychologist to share his or her expert knowledge with others, and shares his from an interest in the possibility of healing. In his interview, he speaks of the psychological damage caused by "suppressed history," and of the freedom that comes with being "no longer burdened" by denial. Having made contact, through a rich series of research studies over the course of his career, with situations of extreme dehumanization, he proceeded to open these situations to the light, via scholarly analysis of the psychology of the survivor, of the perpetrator, and of the atrocity-producing situation. With some similarities to Volkan's work (this volume), Lifton recognizes that the "meaning structures formed by survivors in their death encounter can vary" (Chapter 9), taking forms that work either toward or against further violence, and he seeks through scholarly writing and speaking to contribute to our understanding of what makes the difference.

Mary-Joan Gerson (this volume, Chapter 10) describes in her chapter her month-long experience as a visiting lecturer and public health consultant in Namibia. Although her official role was not clinical, she describes drawing repeatedly on her psychoanalytic training and skills. Attuned to "suppressed history" (in Lifton's words, Chapter 9), she wondered about the contribution of a history of apartheid to contemporary problems with father abandonment and domestic violence. Rather than pressing this point when her students rejected it, she strove to maintain her openness both to the presence of other cultural and historical determinants of contemporary problems, and to the possible reasons for people's investment in not talking about apartheid. While tolerating her own feelings of uncertainty and dislocation, and keeping an eye on her own preconceptions, she continually reoriented herself toward listening and exploration; she felt for opportunities to offer interventions her hosts would welcome. In this her experience provides a model for analysts who step outside their comfort zones to make their expertise publicly available.

While our other contributors may have begun as office-based psychoanalysts and ventured from there to engage with trauma in community settings, Nancy Caro Hollander (this volume, Chapter 11) began as a social historian and was moved through her exposure to state terror, and its psychological effects, into an engagement with psychoanalysis. Her chapter traces her path toward the conclusion that psychoanalysis and politics are meant for one another. Prior to her psychoanalytic training, she felt impelled by the "ethical obligation to raise consciousness" about the human rights violations she had seen as a researcher and activist in Argentina (Chapter 11). She describes being traumatized, without knowing it, by the violence she was witness to, and feeling alienated from and enraged by colleagues who seemed to choose to ignore it. In interviewing survivors of torture, she came to recognize that she lacked the necessary explanatory framework for processing what she heard, a framework her psychoanalytic training would later provide. She learned from Marie Langer of an applied psychoanalytic and political practice that involved offering clinical services to the poor and victimized, training and supervising mental health workers in an impoverished nation, and impromptu therapeutic encounters with workers in factory hallways, with careful management of transference and countertransference dynamics throughout. In ultimately finding her own niche as a critical psychoanalytic scholar, Hollander came to experience first-hand the "reparative healing in the experience of being heard and of finding resonance among colleagues whose preoccupations mirror my own" (Chapter 11).

Elizabeth Hegeman's chapter (Chapter 12) describes the role of activist psychoanalysts in challenging what she frames as the institutional betrayal of its membership by the American Psychological Association (APA). Her analysis of the prolonged battle to have the APA take and enforce a stand against the participation of psychologists in prisoner interrogations both employs psychoanalytic concepts to understand the dynamics of the betrayal involved, and highlights the characteristics of psychoanalysts which uniquely suited them to lead the fight against it. She suggests that longstanding denial and dissociation regarding the APA's institutional misconduct fit the pattern of "blindness" to relational trauma in general, which is adopted as a "coping strategy required for preservation of the relationship" (Chapter 12). She further acknowledges "the pull to dissociate from knowledge that contradicts existing power structures." By way of explaining what enabled many psychoanalysts to resist this pull in the APA's case, Hegeman cites psychoanalysts' clinical experiences with torture survivors, their professional dedication "to thinking about and noticing unconscious and disavowed aggression," and their habituation to "listening for the hidden story" (Reisner, quoted in Chapter 12) "without turning away from unbearable details" (Boulanger, quoted in Chapter 12). Equipped with these tools, psychoanalysts were able repeatedly to speak out against the ethical transgressions they perceived, and ultimately to join in a healing community of those who shared their concerns. In analyzing this painful history, Hegeman promotes an understanding of unconscious motivations and group behavior that, rather than passing blame and polarizing antagonistic sides, seeks to humanize all involved. In a similar spirit to that of Bassin's Combat Paper installation (Chapter 7), her analysis works to foster the acknowledgment of collective responsibility.

In his commentary on Goren and Alpert's interview with Robert Jay Lifton (Chapter 9), Lewis Aron (this volume, Chapter 13) critically examines the postwar social forces that contributed to psychoanalysts' adopting a narrow clinical focus and eschewing politics, an inherently conservative stance. He highlights Lifton's heterodox impulses, in the context of psychoanalytic ideology and training practices that could, at the time of Lifton's training, be rigid and totalizing. Finally, by way of launching readers in the direction of a possible future, he draws our attention to recent movements in psychoanalysis toward increased openness and pluralism, and challenges psychoanalytic institutes to make changes that would have encouraged a candidate like Lifton to stay.

In summary: Adapting the psychoanalytic frame

The expansion of psychoanalysis beyond one-on-one, office-based treatment is motivated by recognition of the many suffering individuals and communities for whom traditional forms of treatment are inaccessible, and by recognition of the unique skills and expertise that psychoanalysis contributes toward the healing of traumas, both individual and collective. The chapters in this book collectively convey the importance of testimony and witnessing, of the establishment of safe, containing spaces, of reconnection with community, and of activism and advocacy in recovery from trauma. Being heard and recognized by one empathic listener may be enough to restore a trauma survivor's sense of being human among humans. Making contact with a community of survivors can have a parallel effect. In the case of collective or shared traumas, engagement in a collective mourning process may be both economical and essential. In light of this, contributors to this volume provide invaluable insights into the nature of collective mourning processes, what inhibits them, and what can move them forward. Psychoanalytic community work can also take the form of scholarship, activism, and advocacy, wherein psychoanalyst writers and speakers expand their purview beyond the psyche and intersubjective relationships of the individual survivor (or community of survivors) to reflect on the ways these are structured by wider social institutions and political ideologies. In this work, too, analysts strive to make the unconscious conscious, and to put disavowed experiences and processes into words.

What skills and perspectives do psychoanalysts uniquely bring to community trauma work? Psychoanalysts bring attunement to the flow of feelings and anxieties—conscious and unconscious, their own and their interlocutors'—over the course of conversations, whether spontaneous or bounded by a clinical frame (Altman). They privilege a stance of inquiry, rather than certainty (Gerson), which opens them to getting to know traumatized people and recognizing their individual responses and needs (Wagner). Psychoanalysts are trained in listening for what is unsaid, for unconscious motivations (Volkan); in metabolizing horrific stories and painful affects without themselves disavowing or dissociating what they hear (Hegeman); and in attending to the dynamic sequelae of past traumas as these emerge in current relationships. Psychoanalysts are trained in representing what they have heard both in and under the surface of others' words, in helping to make others' feelings and experiences thinkable, speakable, and portrayable (Ainslie, Bassin). Telling one's story in the presence of such a listener can facilitate reengagement with disavowed feelings and experiences, and can enable frozen grief to thaw and mourning to proceed (Laub). Whatever else may change when psychoanalysts work in non-traditional settings, therefore, Nina Thomas (Foreword, this volume) reminds us "not to alter the quality of listening we bring."

The contributors to this volume have together shown us a wealth of possibilities in the diverse kinds of work analysts can do once we expand our analytic identities (see Introduction, this volume) and choose, judiciously, to open our office doors. The editors of this volume argue that these attitudes of expansion and openness are crucial to the continued health and continuing growth of psychoanalysis. To move into the future, psychoanalysis must embrace its pre-World War II past, and become once again more widely available and more progressively involved, acknowledging and applying itself to the social issues of our day. The work described here amply demonstrates that psychoanalytic training confers key skills and techniques of great utility to practitioners of applied, socially engaged interventions. All the same, expanding their purviews to include community work will pose challenges to traditionally trained analysts. To bring their skills to bear where they are most needed, psychoanalysts will need to be willing to redefine the analytic frame, and to relinquish the relative security and control the office setting and the highly structured, one-on-one, therapeutic relationship afford.

A number of our contributors (Altman, Boulanger, Roth) have testified to the unease and uncertainty analysts can experience when working in unconventional or unstable settings. At the same time, as Altman (this volume) points out, the analytic frame may itself be a culture-bound construct, most comfortable to those of Northern European/North American (and it may be, upper-middle class) backgrounds, and potentially experienced as destabilizing by patients from elsewhere. What aspects of the analytic frame, then, can be sacrificed to the good, and what aspects are essential to psychoanalysis and must be retained? Privacy and anonymity will each to some degree be compromised during many forms of community work. Engaging in community-based work will often require us to be prepared to share more of ourselves, whether it be personal information, food, or our visible presence in public places. It will require that we let ourselves be known, while remaining ever mindful of transference and countertransference issues. As the face of psychoanalysis becomes more publicly visible, analysts will necessarily become less like blank slates and more "real," both to the people we are helping and to the other people, both professional and non-professional, who will inevitably be simultaneously involved. Such collaborative encounters have the potential to be highly productive, if we dare to venture out toward them.

Challenges involved in creating a modified, "portable" analytic frame include establishing an appropriate psychological distance, maintaining ethical boundaries, and otherwise promoting the psychological safety of those with whom we intervene. In order to preserve these essential elements under non-standardized conditions, we will need to learn new methods for building a frame around each therapeutic encounter that is sensitive to the specificity and uniqueness of each situation. Locating the ideal psychological distance poses challenges even in conventional treatment and becomes even more challenging when one moves beyond the confines of the office into complex social and physical environments, such as those described in the chapters above. One must find a position that is neither removed to the point of irrelevance nor over-involved to the point of being counterproductive. In the interests of maintaining ethical boundaries in newly unbounded relationships, we will need to remember that there is a distinct difference between a therapeutic interaction and a contract to engage in therapy, and that some of our most treasured ways of working may be out of place in the absence of such a contract. For example, although interpretations can and should inform an analyst's actions, explicitly rendering an interpretation is often not appropriate in community-based work.

Precisely because there is so much to learn, the foundations for the expansion of psychoanalysis into socially engaged community work will necessarily be laid in the psychoanalytic training institutes. This will require some adjustment and expansion of psychoanalytic curricula. For example, new courses could focus on preparing candidates to work in mental health disaster relief (as in Chapter 3), or to work in chaotic, uncontrolled, or unstable environments (as in Chapter 5), or with less familiar populations. Candidates will need to be prepared to engage in professional collaborations with non-analysts, and to introduce themselves into settings where their own professional expertise may not be immediately recognized. More consideration will have to be given to cultural differences, as well as to social and political issues as these impact our patients' mental health. As Aron notes (this volume, Chapter 13), "[e]ven now, and even in New York City, how much attention is being paid in psychoanalytic institutes to such practical matters as poverty, homelessness, immigration, the devastation of the union movement, nuclear threat, and political oppression?" Adapting Hollander (Chapter 11), "the customary emphasis on the familial-based etiology of psychological disorders [must] be situated in the larger social context of ideological and institutional structuring of unconscious processes and intersubjective experience."

We will end by raising the question at the back of everyone's mind: Is this really psychoanalysis? There are those who will argue that thinking of these kinds of interventions as analytic dilutes the concept, or the "purity," of psychoanalysis. But what is psychoanalysis if not whatever a trained psychoanalyst does in the service of bearing witness, striving to alleviate suffering, and helping people make sense of the world in which they are living, the life they have lived, and their possible futures? The contributors to this volume have posed a challenge to psychoanalytic orthodoxy by bringing their clinical skills, theoretical understanding, and sense of responsibility as "citizen analysts" to bear on socio-political conflicts and other catastrophic situations. Lest you think this is heresy, let us remind you that 50 years ago, Erich Fromm, who was known for the one session treatment, made the argument that psychoanalysis is defined by an attempt to help the patient by means of understanding the unconscious. And finally, almost 100 years ago, Freud defined psychoanalysis thus:

> ...Psychoanalysis is an attempt to account for two striking and unexpected facts ... the facts of transference and of resistance. Any line of investigation which recognizes these two facts and takes them as the starting-point of its work has a right to call itself psycho-analysis.
>
> (1914, p. 16)

References

Brothers, D. (2009). Trauma-Centered Psychoanalysis: Transforming Experiences of Unbearable Uncertainty. *Self and Systems: Annals of the New York Academy of Sciences, 1159*, pp. 51–62.

Freud, S. (1914). On the history of the psycho-analytic movement. In *The Standard Edition of the Complete Psychological Works of Sigmund Freud, Vol. 14*. Translated and edited by J. Strachey. London: Hogarth Press, 1957, pp. 1–66.

Goren, E. (2011). *Beyond the Reach of Ladders: My Story as a Therapist Forging Bonds with Firefighters in the Aftermath of 9/11*. London: Open Gate Press.

Herman, J. (1992). *Trauma and Recovery: The Aftermath of Violence, from Domestic Abuse to Political Terror.* New York, NY: Basic Books.

Levy, M.A., Haglund, P., Plaut, L., Emde, R., Stewart, M., Shaw, R., et al. (2004). Healing After Columbine: Reflections of Psychoanalytic Responders to Community Trauma. *Journal of the American Psychoanalytic Association, 52*(3), pp. 759–781.

Index